Praise for

THE
ALKALINE RESET CLEANSE

"*The Alkaline Reset Cleanse* is a new way of thinking about your body, and it rocks. Ross will show you how to use the healing power of nature and your intuition—no starving, no cravings, nothing like your typical 'detox.' Radiant health is possible; let this wonderful book guide the way."

— **Kris Carr**, *New York Times* best-selling author

"The body is out of balance, the immune system is compromised, and the resulting environment is perfect for disease creation. Ross Bridgeford addresses both of these root causes (deficiency and toxicity) in his groundbreaking book, *The Alkaline Reset Cleanse*. It's a simple, easy-to-follow guide that can teach you how to take control of your own health and literally activate your body's self-healing mechanism and create an internal environment that fosters health rather than sickness. My recommendation is simple: Buy this book."

— **Ty M. Bollinger**, documentary film producer and best-selling author of
The Truth about Cancer

"*The Alkaline Reset Cleanse* isn't just another diet or detox. It's a road map for how to be super healthy and prosper at every level—physically, mentally, and emotionally. This is the ultimate guide for super vitality and total mind-body health."

— **Jon Gabriel**, creator of The Gabriel Method and best-selling author
of *Visualization for Weight Loss*

"I so enjoyed this book! It totally satisfied the science geek in me who has been curious for years about the whole 'alkaline diet' thing. Whether you're in a health crisis and desperately need an emergency overhaul or are humming along and just want some powerful health hacks to add to your regimen, *The Alkaline Reset Cleanse* will deliver the goods."

— **Susan Peirce Thompson, Ph.D.**, *New York Times* best-selling author of
Bright Line Eating

"Ross has done an amazing job of simplifying exactly how to raise our energy without relying on quick fixes that leave us feeling even worse. Instead, he provides a science-backed blueprint, helping you raise your energy naturally and quickly so that you live your life to the fullest. Read this book, apply its simple principles, and watch how your body and energy transform."

— **Yuri Elkaim**, *New York Times* best-selling author of *The All-Day Energy Diet*

"There is no one I trust more when it comes to sharing alkaline science in an approachable way than Ross Bridgeford. *The Alkaline Reset Cleanse* simplifies the alkaline diet so that people can succeed. There are so many fad diets out there, and they all lead to deprivation. That's not sustainable. Ross's approach fits into anyone's life, no matter where they're starting from or what their goals are. Ross is a master at showing you how to reset your health and make progress toward a life filled with health and unstoppable energy!"

— **Dr. Daryl Gioffre**, founder and CEO, Gioffre Chiropractic Wellness Center, Alkamind, and author of *Get Off Your Acid*

"Alkalizing your diet can completely transform your life, and this book will show you how."

— **James Colquhoun**, filmmaker of *Food Matters* and *Hungry for Change* and founder of FMTV

THE
ALKALINE RESET CLEANSE

THE
ALKALINE RESET CLEANSE

The 7-Day Reboot for Unlimited Energy, Rapid Weight
Loss, and the Prevention of Degenerative Disease

ROSS BRIDGEFORD

HAY HOUSE, INC.
Carlsbad, California • New York City
London • Sydney • New Delhi

Copyright © 2018 by Ross Bridgeford

Published in the United States by: Hay House, Inc.: www.hayhouse.com® • **Published in Australia by:** Hay House Australia Pty. Ltd.: www.hayhouse.com.au • **Published in the United Kingdom by:** Hay House UK, Ltd.: www.hayhouse.co.uk • **Published in India by:** Hay House Publishers India: www.hayhouse.co.in

Indexer: Joan Shapiro
Cover and interior design: Nick C. Welch

Cataloging-in-Publication Data is on file with the Library of Congress

Hardcover ISBN: 978-1-4019-5548-9
e-book ISBN: 978-1-4019-5549-6

10 9 8 7 6 5 4 3 2 1
1st edition, December 2018

Printed in the United States of America

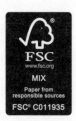
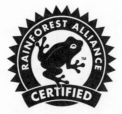

To Tania,
Leo & Joe

CONTENTS

FOREWORD

What you're about to learn from Ross Bridgeford has never been more important.

It is no secret that we're facing a health crisis, and that it's reaching epidemic proportions. Obesity, heart disease, type 2 diabetes, cancer, Alzheimer's, and autoimmune diseases like arthritis have reached frightening levels. For all the billions of dollars we're spending on diet books and programs, and for all the trillions we're spending on high-tech medical interventions, most people just keep getting fatter and sicker.

What's driving this cycle of disease?

It's the food.

Research has proven that the number-one factor fueling our epidemic of degenerative disease is the modern diet. From digestive complaints and reflux to conditions such as rheumatoid arthritis, Hashimoto's thyroiditis, and so much more, the food we eat is promoting sickness and suffering.

If your arteries become so clogged that you die, you might see "heart attack" listed as the cause of death. But the truth is, heart attack won't really be the cause of death. It will have been a diet and lifestyle that made a heart attack predictable.

The major illnesses of our times aren't actually causes of death—they're symptoms. The modern diet is creating an environment that sets the stage for sickness and disease to be almost inevitable.

So what the heck should you eat?

Everybody and their brother has an opinion. We hear that fat is bad, then we hear that it's the best way to stay thin. We hear that coconut oil is a magic cure-all for everything, and then we hear that it's poisonous. We hear that animal products cause heart disease, and then we hear that butter and bacon are back. Your acupuncturist, your naturopath, and your opinionated aunt all give you different advice. And chances are, your doctor acts as if what you eat hardly matters at all.

Today we have access to billions of web pages, tens of thousands of books, and hundreds of thousands of so-called experts offering nutritional insights and information.

Unfortunately, they all seem to point in different directions. And many of them are wrong.

In a sea of confusion, the status quo prevails. Unfortunately—even tragically—we all know where that leads.

I don't know the reason you have this book in your hands right now. It could be because you're in a crisis situation, facing a serious diagnosis, or it could be because you want to experience more energy and vitality in your life. But whatever the reason, here's the reality: If you want to thrive, if you want to love your life, if you want a vibrant and fabulous relationship with food and with your body, then you're in the right place.

When Ross told me he was writing this book, I was delighted for two reasons. One, because I know Ross has helped to transform thousands of lives, and I want the whole world to have the benefit of his message.

And secondly, I'm delighted because we need this book now. We need the message it brings, and we need to put it into action. The fundamentals that Ross will teach you could change your health forever.

What you will find within these pages are the simple steps, one day at a time, that Ross has used to help thousands of clients to refresh and restore their bodies.

Yours could be next.

This is not your typical "cleanse" or "detox." It is a whole body reboot—strong enough to help you undo the ravages of the modern diet, and gentle enough to nourish, soothe, and heal you from the inside out.

By focusing on the twin powers of 1) nature and 2) the capacity of your body to heal itself, Ross cuts through the confusion. His guidelines are simple to follow and, most importantly, easy to stick with for the long-term. This is no "quick fix" or "magic bullet" that will fade on the other end to leave you back where you started.

The Alkaline Reset Cleanse will set you solidly on a new path and deliver benefits that can stay with you for a lifetime.

And don't be deceived by the fact that Ross's plan is accessible and easy to follow. What he teaches you is evidence-based and rooted in extensive scientific data. He's done the research and hard work, and has distilled it into the potent plan you now hold in your hands.

And did I mention that this can be fun? Some people fear that eating healthy food will be boring. It's true that the industrialized food industry has done a pretty good job producing the cheapest, tastiest, and most nutritionally inferior food-like products in the history of the world.

But when you base your diet around real, whole, nutrient-dense foods, your taste buds will actually begin to change. Over time, you will find that you grow to love foods that love you back. You may come to experience more pleasure, and more joy, than you ever imagined possible.

Over the course of the next 21 days, you're going to create changes in your body. And your body just might thank you for the rest of your life.

Food is deeply personal—and it's also political. It changes your life, and it changes your world. By following the Alkaline Reset Cleanse, you will start a powerful ripple effect. You will be starting a mini-Food Revolution of your own.

Your choices at your local grocery store, with your family, at social gatherings, and with your friends and workmates will all create a positive influence. And when people in your world see the vitality radiating from every cell in your body, they too might want to learn more and to start their own journey.

The book you hold in your hands is a key to a new way of eating and a new way of living. You'll be joining in one of the most important movements of our times—a Food Revolution that is literally shifting the course of history.

Welcome.

Ocean Robbins, November 2018
Author of *31-Day Food Revolution*
Founder, Food Revolution Network
www.foodrevolution.org

INTRODUCTION

I'm so excited you've joined me on this journey. It's quick, but the results are lifelong. It's simple, but it brings about complex changes inside your body on a cellular level. It's painless, but it kick-starts a powerful transformation. Whether you struggle with weight, inflammation, chronic fatigue or pain, adrenal or thyroid imbalances, digestive issues, high blood pressure, type 2 diabetes, or gout, or whether you just want more energy, confidence in your body, better sleep, greater strength, or mental clarity, rest assured that the guidance in this book will help you.

The Alkaline Reset Cleanse (ARC) gets to the root causes and puts your body into a state where it can heal, rebuild, replenish, and thrive. I have coached thousands upon thousands of people to amazing health with the ARC, and you will be inspired by some of their stories throughout this book.

The first success story I want to share with you, though, isn't about someone who lost 100 pounds or shrank a brain tumor on my plan (both of which I have seen happen). It's the story of a stressed-out new parent who had lost his way with his health, barely slept, gained weight, struggled to focus, felt overwhelmed, and couldn't seem to get out from under the pressure of life.

That new dad was me.

During the summer my first son was born, my health had reached a breaking point. I'd moved countries and then cities (twice). My partner, Tania, and I had just knocked down a house to build a new one. I'd walked away from a business partnership to start another from scratch. And if all that wasn't enough, we faced the biggest challenge of all, the arrival of our new baby boy, Leo.

His birth was the most incredible moment of my life (now shared with the birth of our second child, Joe) but, wow, my already very maxed-out life suddenly got a whole lot busier. Juggling as much as I could, I fell into the all-too-common trap of putting my health last. I had a big bag of excuses ready, like, "I don't have time for a run" or "I've got to get to the office, but I'll make a juice later." The run and the juice? Never happened.

At first, the decline of my health was gradual. I started to feel tired more often, but I put it down to working long hours or a bad night's sleep. (Leo was not a great sleeper, to put it mildly.) My weight ticked up, but I told myself I didn't have as much time to exercise, I'd get back to the gym "tomorrow." My digestion flared with on-and-off shooting pains throughout the day, but I was sure it was the stress of the business and eating on the run.

When Leo was six months old, every symptom I'd been experiencing doubled, then rapidly tripled. It was a do-or-die situation. If I didn't get it rocking and rolling to support my new family, I wouldn't be able to give them everything I wanted them to have. So I worked harder, grinding on all cylinders, but I still didn't seem to be getting anywhere.

For months, I'd wake up in the middle of the night in panic mode, unable to sleep, ruminating on every worst-case scenario, and convincing myself that doom was inevitable.

I just felt so trapped and hopeless. When I went deep into my anxiety—that I'd never be enough, that I was a failure, that I'd let my family down and be a terrible example to my newborn son—I could feel a knot forming in my core, tightening nonstop, growing every day.

I felt too exhausted to be the father I wanted to be, to be a good partner in my relationship, or to make my new business a success. I felt like I was letting everyone down. More than anything, I just wanted to know my family was happy, and that my son would respect me and look back on his childhood with fondness about the time we spent together and the life I was able to give him.

The situation just kept spiraling downward, and might have continued forever if it weren't for Tania, my angel. Even though I never talk about my problems—I'm more the silent type who bottles things up—she saw the pain and stress in my eyes. Tania sat me down and laid out some harsh truths. By working myself into the ground and putting off my health until "tomorrow," I was doing the opposite of what I intended, which was to support and protect my family. I feel blessed to have someone close to me who wasn't afraid to tell it like it was. It changed the course of my life for good.

One of my main issues, as I eventually came to understand, was that I was being ruled by my fear. Fear of failure for one. Even more, I believe a fear of *success* was holding me back. What if I succeeded and got into the perfect state of health and removed all the roadblocks, and turned out to be a lousy dad? What if I reached my health goals but I *still* was not reaching my business goals?

When I told people about this, they were surprised at first, but then they often said, "Actually, I know what you mean. Fear has held me back, too. I worry that if I get healthy, my family and friends will judge me, won't be happy for me, or they'll stop wanting to hang out with me if I'm not drinking or if I'm being healthy all of the time."

Once I got a handle on the emotional piece, I turned toward the physical problem. Part of my frustration was that I already had the answers about how to get healthy and in shape again. After all, my life leading up to this had been characterized by my full health—I had been absolutely rocking it, thriving, and running marathons, on top of everything else. However, now that I was in my 30s, the things I did in my 20s didn't seemed to be working. My attempts to go cold turkey on everything "bad" were completely unrealistic and unachievable. Throwing supplements at the problem didn't seem to work like it used to.

I needed to stop, step back, and sort this whole thing out. There had to be a solution to my problem for the way I lived *now*. My health was getting beyond that and the stress, busy-ness, lack of time—my standby excuses—were getting the better of me.

The very first step to rebuilding my life and health was deciding to live by *one important rule* that would direct everything I did: My family and my health are the most important things in my life. Everything had to start from this one foundational rule.

I swore on that day that never again, ever, would anything compromise either my health or my family. I set about reorganizing my life to assert my priorities. Instead of obsessing about work and success, I took time out. Instead of fixating on the bottom line, I invested in my health again.

Does this ring any bells for you? When people tell me about their stumbles into ill health, I can only nod in agreement, because it's been my path, too. We've all faced the struggles, challenges, and frustrations of getting (re)started and making it stick, only to be disappointed and frustrated over and over again.

My personal journey through frustration, fear, and disappointment is the reason the Alkaline Reset Cleanse exists. If I hadn't gotten to such a desperate place, I wouldn't have been inspired to create the program to heal myself, and then, others. If I didn't have a personal stake in the ARC's ability to heal, I would not have been so ardent in my research.

You Can Transform Your Health

I've been coaching people to reach their biggest health goals for over 15 years, but since I created the Alkaline Reset Cleanse as a full online program, my clients have achieved a whole new level of results. I've now guided more than 9,000 people through the process with a 100 percent success rate among the 92 percent who completed the program.

I designed the Cleanse to be simple, using ordinary kitchen equipment and delicious food you can buy in any supermarket. You won't starve yourself (more like the opposite!), and my clients all report that the plan is enjoyable to follow. From Day One, they see and *feel* the results, which makes it fun, exciting, and a pleasure to continue. There is almost nothing in the world that would make you want to stop feeling this good.

Why does one program work so well across the board for all different kinds of people in various states of health? Of course, we each have individual genetics, a dietary history that is unique, and our own reason for needing to reset our body. But as different as we are, we share the same basic biology. We all have the same systems, hormones, and organs. We also share the same environment, diet, and culture that cause the health conditions and problems we face, and the ARC gets to the core of what the human body needs to reset, rebalance, and put you in the optimal state to thrive.

The ARC is not your normal detox, reboot, or cleanse. In fact, most people are shocked at how pain-free and easy it is. I worked continuously to refine and improve it to what it is today. This is my life mission. Nothing is as gratifying to me personally as watching people do the plan I've been perfecting for so long and knowing that their lives are about to change.

To turn my health around, and ultimately to create what has become the ARC, I sought out trained experts—dozens of doctors, research scientists, and specialists in completely different areas of expertise from mine—to work and brainstorm with me. I have been known as the "alkaline diet guy" for over a decade, but their expertise in areas such as hormonal imbalance, autoimmune conditions, gut health, insulin resistance and diabetes, metabolism, blood, stress, and the brain, complemented everything I had been researching and teaching. These additional layers took my coaching and the results I was getting for my clients to a whole new level. And boy, I studied voraciously. Suddenly I was going so much deeper than just our pH balance. While it was clear that our pH was still at the root of everything—ensuring your body maintains its alkaline balance is absolutely essential—I now understood it was so inter-related with our other body systems in ways I had never realized before. And when you overlay these other systems with your body's pH balance, everything suddenly becomes so much more powerful and the path to incredible health becomes so clear.

Over the course of study, I realized that my curiosity about the human body was boundless and that I had a knack for deciphering and extrapolating data. (I'm a total science geek, but I always keep the info simple for you!)

Study after study, expert after expert, I followed the common thread toward a solution. One thing kept coming through, over and over again. It emerged so strongly, it was like a slap in the face.

That one recurring theme was *balance.*

I'm not talking about "work-life balance." Although it is important, and I'd certainly suffered from an imbalance there, it only scratched the surface. The key to health and energy is for your body's intricately connected systems to be in balance, a.k.a. *homeostasis.* Whether it's your pH, hormones, digestion, weight, brain, liver, kidneys, heart, or anything else in between, if one particu-lar system or organ is out of whack, everything will fall apart. You have to treat the whole to heal the parts.

Every minute of every day, your body is working *so* hard to maintain homeostasis, or to return to it. Balance is the overarching, single most important goal of your body. When any of your body's thousands of delicate balances—hormone, gut bacteria, white and red blood cell production, enzymes, immune system, pH, to mention a few—are off, sickness, disease, fatigue, weight gain, and pain are the inevitable result.

Our stressful lives, lack of sleep, and the standard Western diet—sugar, soda, alcohol, takeout, and processed foods—are all constantly pulling our bodies away from balance and forcing them to fight their way back.

But what if we provided ourselves with the nourishment needed to main-tain balance effortlessly? We would unclog, reset, and *thrive.*

When I built the nutritional plan to flood my body and cells with exactly what they needed to heal and repair, my health and my life turned around rap-idly. Through a long process of trial and error, I hit upon a protocol that kept me satisfied and full and wasn't hard at all to do, and it put my body back into balance. Almost immediately:

- My skin, which had returned to being spotty and pale like when I was a teen, became totally clear again.

- My energy went from rock bottom to sustained and consistently high all day.

- The dangerous layer of visceral fat that had formed (the "skinny fat" tire that is *so* indicative of serious health concerns) melted away.

- My fatigued adrenals bounced back to normal.

- My blood work—LDL, HDL, triglycerides—went from borderline to beautiful. (FYI: In the alkaline world, people have "blood microscopy" work done, or the harvesting of live blood cells to look at them under a microscope. All I could see under the scope were beautiful, round, healthy red blood cells.)

In short, I was back in balance and rocking it.

Perhaps most important, thanks to my restored health, my confidence returned. I felt vibrant and alive, and I was able to contribute to the happiness of my family again. Energy and joy came roaring back, along with patience, calm, and concentration. By fueling my body, I allowed it to rebalance by giving it the nourishment it needed, and I was rewarded with inner calm and positivity that I hadn't felt in a long time.

I could almost sense my life-span lengthening. I could see myself playing with my kids and grandkids (and great-grandkids) for many years to come. If I made it easy for my body to stay in balance, I would have the freedom to move and travel and enjoy my life right up until the day I die.

RESET, REBALANCE, AND RECONNECT

The process of resetting made me aware of how essential it is to appreciate and feel connected to my body. Your body is a miracle, and when you fuel it, nourish it, and love it, it lifts up your whole life. The magic happens when you realize that *you are your body*, and that you need to care for it gently and completely.

Your body knows how to thrive; you just need to give it the tools to do so. Nourishing yourself, nurturing yourself, and focusing on abundance are how you love yourself. These X-factors are sorely missing in trendy "diets," and the reason such plans fail. They emphasize the negatives—"don't," "bad," "restrict"—and pit you *against* your body. They make health and weight loss seem like a fight to the death. If you've bounced from one of those limiting plans to the next, it's no wonder you might see your body as the enemy, or as a disgusting appendage. When I first meet clients, they often tell me, "I hate my body," "I wish I had a different body," "I wish I had a faster metabolism," or "My body puts on weight so easily." Many people live their whole lives as if their bodies are a different entity from themselves.

Your body and your mind are not two separate things. You *are* your body. You and your body are on the same team. As you go through the process in this book, you will learn to work with your body for the greater good and give it exactly what it needs. By loving yourself, your health (and other) goals will be reached. We've worn ourselves out from beating ourselves up.

That's all over now. You are about to love yourself to health and happiness, and it's going to feel *sensational*.

No matter what your goal, the ARC will move you dramatically closer (if not all of the way there) to homeostasis in seven days. Some clients might have gotten into the ARC to lose weight or heal digestive woes, but practically *everyone* gets a whole lot of other surprising bonus results, too, including their allergies disappearing, skin conditions clearing up, having a boost in potency, better sleep, and a positive mood. "I wasn't expecting *that* to happen!" they say. I love that aspect of the plan. When you're restored, balanced, and reconnected with yourself, joyful surprises are to be expected.

EVERYTHING YOU NEED IS ALREADY INSIDE YOU, AND ON THESE PAGES

By now, I hope you're excited to get started.

As you read on, keep in mind the one overriding principle behind the ARC: harnessing the power of nature. You will use simple, real, whole, natural foods and trust in your body's natural healing ability to fix itself. You won't rely on products, pills, powders, or supplements here, nor insta-cures or magic bullets. I do recommend a few supplements, but they are only extra doses of nature's goodness that act as a backup.

On this Earth, we have been given all the tools we need to thrive, and on the ARC, you will use and embrace them. When you leverage the power of nature, you'll see not only how amazing it is, but also how simple it *should be* to have a life of abundant health, all-day energy, and freedom from pain, sickness, and disease. During the seven days of the Cleanse, you will feel light, energized, positive, and excited. One of my most favorite pieces of feedback from clients is that they feel *joy* during the Cleanse. Just like it did for me, the ARC will give you an abundance of confidence—and not just confidence in how you feel and what you see when you stand in front of the mirror. It will give you a confidence that runs a level deeper, so that your body can stay healthy, fit, strong, and vital for decades to come.

Right now, take a moment to pause. Close your eyes and think about your biggest, wildest health goal. Picture what that looks like. Imagine a scene playing out with you in it, inside your ideal body with your dream health and vitality, and the energy, strength, and confidence you'll feel.

It is within reach.

You already have everything you need to get started, but first, I want to give you a quick overview of what you'll find in this book and *why* you are practically guaranteeing success for yourself.

I've organized the book into three main parts:

Part I is a brief dive into the nature of the beast, in other words, why people's health falters, and why our culture and environment make it hard to stay healthy. What are the root causes of ill health? Why are we facing particular challenges right now? In this section, you'll become a student again, and learn (unlearn, relearn) about your body. Don't worry! No pop quizzes here. Just some basic insight into your body's Five Master Systems (which are responsible for 95 percent of your health) and the three main causes of disease. Then I'll explain how to turn things around, namely with my Triple A Method to restoring health.

Part II digs into the Alkaline Reset Cleanse: what it is, how it works, why it works, and what it looks like. I'll go over the Five Pillars of the ARC, and give you a breakdown of the types of foods and recipes you'll be eating and drinking, the nutrient profile of a day on the Cleanse, the equipment you'll need, what the Cleanse will be doing in your body, and *why it works so amazingly well for so many different health goals.* By the end of Part II, you'll have a comprehensive understanding of the logistics, mechanics, and philosophy of the Cleanse—and you'll feel incredibly motivated to jump right in!

Finally, **Part III** is the day-by-day, step-by-step breakdown of doing the Cleanse. It has three phases: the week before, the week during, and the rest of your life after. You will have the complete blueprint, along with shopping lists, recipes, advice, and encouragement to see you through easily, enjoyably, and effortlessly.

There is no guesswork here. If you follow the steps, you will get results.

So let's do this!

PART I

THE NATURE OF THE BEAST

CHAPTER 1

HOW DID WE GET HERE?

We know more about the human body now than at any other point in history. We have an intricate understanding of practically every tiny process. We know exactly how the body works, why it works, what it needs, what makes it tick, and what makes it sick.

Yet cancer rates are skyrocketing.

Obesity is at a crisis point. It's getting worse every year, and the pace is accelerating at an alarming rate.

Diet-related illness is costing the United States economy more than $1.3 *trillion* every year,[1] and if it continues at this rate, it will hit $4.2 trillion in 2023. In other words, the economy is going to implode.

Heads are firmly in the sand. The entire situation is a slow-motion train wreck on a global scale that we all know is happening, but hardly anything is being done to stop it.

It has reached crisis level. *The worldwide community is eating itself to death.* Almost 70 percent of the U.S. population is overweight; shockingly, 38 percent of adults and 20 percent of children are obese. Not just overweight, but obese. This figure is predicted to hit 50 percent just after 2020.[2] What's more, 35 percent of the population has type 2 diabetes or are prediabetic.[3] As of July 2017, that translates to almost 100 million people in the U.S. who are sick and getting sicker.

This just isn't sustainable. We all know something has to change, but before that can happen, we have to understand how we got here.

And before we get into that, it is important for you to understand:

It's not your fault.

No matter your situation right now, whether you consider your health an 8 out of 10 and want to take it to the top notch or if you're a 1 out of 10 and desperate to change, the odds have been stacked against you.

The media, official government guidelines, (most) doctors and physicians, food manufacturing and marketing companies, supermarkets and grocery stores, and quick-fix diet trends have completely led you in the wrong direction.

In so many cases, what they've all told you is the exact opposite of what you should be doing. Magazines just need a new diet to put on the covers every month, regardless of whether it "works" or is safe. Doctors are "encouraged" by Big Pharma to treat with prescriptions. Big Food companies and supermarkets want to sell you the cheapest food at the highest prices.

Meanwhile, say you're a working mom with three kids and you want to give your family the best food you can on your budget, so you buy "whole wheat" pasta, tomato sauce, and "part-skim" cheese. And since you're all in such a hurry in the morning, you give your kids "heart-healthy" cereals and skim milk. As I'll get into in later chapters, cheese and milk, especially the "skim" varieties, are actually harmful for growing bones. Many things you've been led to believe are good for your family's health are the opposite.

Considering the confusion and conflicting info out there, and the fact that life often gets in the way of good health, I wouldn't be surprised at all that any health challenge you might be dealing with right now might seem overwhelming. You might add insult to injury by blaming, shaming, and guilting yourself, which only makes you feel worse and makes it harder to lose weight or get better (stress hormones increase belly fat; you can't worry yourself thin).

You've been let down by misinformation, over and over. If you haven't been able to reach your health goals, I'll say it again, *it's not your fault.*

I've been coaching and teaching this stuff for almost 15 years, guiding my clients away from sickness, toward radiant health. Even today, the people who join the online program for the Alkaline Reset Cleanse, and those who join me in my coaching membership (The Alkaline Base Camp) are shocked when they hear about these health lies. They feel let down and frustrated that they've been sold this misinformation for so many years.

But the good news is that regardless of where your health is now or how hard you've tried and failed to change in the past, you can turn things around.

The solution is simple. No matter your starting place, we are going to get you incredible results.

Forgive yourself. Shake off any negative emotions about how your health got out of hand. It's not your fault, and you're already taking control by reading this book.

Now let's get to work sorting it all out.

The Three Causes of Our Collective Health Crisis

You can probably already guess the three main causes of our collective health crisis.

1. Big Food Marketing

If you distrust Big Pharma (which you possibly *should*), then you should also have healthy skepticism about Big Food manufacturing marketing. Big Foods are the megabrands of fast, packaged, and refined foods found in the middle aisles of the supermarket (the stuff in a colorful box or crinkly plastic wrapper) and any fast-food chain restaurant.

Most people don't actively distrust these companies, and certainly aren't wary of Keebler Elves and Tony the Tiger. After all, most people have been eating Big Food their whole lives. They have happy childhood memories about Lucky Charms and Ritz crackers. But just because you've always done something does not mean you should keep on doing it.

Start your reeducation about health by asking, "What is the number-one goal of the Big Food businesses?" Is it your health or their bottom line?

Ninety-nine percent of Big Food manufacturing companies (such as Coca-Cola, Mars, General Mills, McDonald's, Nestlé) operate with one guiding goal: to get you addicted to their products so you buy as much and as frequently as possible. As long as you're buying, they don't give a damn whether their products are good. Correction: They don't care if their products are destroying your health. They spend billions to create foods that are the perfect blend of salt,[1] sugar, unhealthy fat, and man-made chemicals so that it's practically *impossible* to eat just one. It's a formula, a recipe for addiction. They've cracked the code, and they know exactly what they're doing in creating it.

---

1   I'm certainly not saying all salt is bad (some is very, very good for you and absolutely necessary), but these companies' use of sodium chloride (refined table salt) with these other ingredients is proven to make their products addictive.

If they were making really tasty treats that were only *theoretically* addictive, say, *by accident*, then why use ingredients like monosodium glutamate (MSG) and aspartame, known carcinogens and hormone disruptors? They pour those in with a heavy hand because they are proven to be physically and chemically addictive, lighting up the pleasure center in the brain like a Christmas tree. You want to feel that high again, so you have another bag of chips or a bowl of cereal. Junk food is a very powerful drug. Sugar is like cocaine.[4] The foods these companies make contain just the right combination of ingredients to get you hooked and craving more.

It's not fair and it's not pretty. Junk-food cravings and addictions are happening every day to millions and millions of people.

The deception doesn't end with the ingredients list. Big Food is sneaky. These companies leverage government guidelines to disguise their products in packaging lies. For example, the lie that kept lying for 30 years found on Big Food in nearly every aisle of the supermarket, was the claim that "low-fat" or "lite" foods were healthy. Nothing could be further from the truth!

But if they say it's true, most people automatically believe it, naturally assuming there is truth in advertising or that government agencies would crack down on false claims. For decades, the scientific community has known that *sugar* is the culprit when it comes to weight gain, diabetes, cancer, and heart disease—*not fat*. Research has shown for years that fat is not the culprit and is absolutely vital for human health.[5]

But Big Food companies continue to push "low-fat" foods as saviors because they're cheaper to make, easy to make delicious (just add lots of sugar or chemical sugar substitutes), and easier to premium price. The reality is, low-fat foods are absolutely devastating to your body. They are, without exception, loaded with sugar and stuffed with carcinogenic, inflammatory, hormone-disrupting chemicals. But *somehow* they are allowed to be called "healthy" and get that government stamp of approval.

Another scam: It's been known for years that gluten-containing grains (wheat, rye, barley, and spelt) are inflammatory, damage the brain,[6] and cause insulin resistance,[7] leaky gut, and many more conditions. However, "whole-grain" foods are touted as being healthy. Big Food manufacturers love to slap that message on any product that is cheap to produce and easy to premium price and sell to people who believe in them.

Suffice it to say, your health and well-being are at the murky bottom of Big Food's priority list.

2. The Need for Speed

Our super-busy, always-rushing culture demands that we search for quick answers to problems, even if the problem is, "What's for breakfast/lunch/dinner?" We love to hit the fast-and-easy button or swallow the magic pill. We're more crazed, stressed, and time-poor than at any other time in history.

Most of us stock the freezer with prepackaged food, load up a takeout box from a hot buffet, order in, or eat out. Who's got time to cook from scratch, let alone shop for fresh ingredients?

But "I'm too busy to cook" is the collective lie we've told ourselves (some more than others, myself included) over the past 40 years. Our grandparents, even our parents, managed to cook dinner every night, and they didn't have many of the time-saving conveniences we do now. The reality is, it takes the same amount of time to go to the grocery store and buy and cook mac and cheese as it does to stock up on fresh veggies and chop them into a salad. (Really. I've timed it.) But we still live under the delusion that cooking is a chore and takes forever.

When we say "yes" to convenience, and "no" to cooking, we wind up eating the processed, refined, and preserved foods that make us fat and sick. Microwaved meals, jars of sauce, breads, pastas, fast food, takeaways, baked goods, ready meals . . . 99 percent of them are packed with the most acid-forming, inflammatory ingredients you can find: sugar, gluten, MSG, chemicals, sweeteners, colorings, flavorings, trans fats, hydrogenated fats, and high-fructose corn syrup, all with zero nutritional value. And that's just scratching the surface. They also clog your digestive system, disrupt practically every hormone in your body, stress the liver, create chronic acidosis, expedite the production of fat cells, weaken the immune system, and so much more.

Not only that, but while you impoverish your body of nutrients, you're enriching Big Food profit margins. Double whammy.

3. The Rapid Rise in Sugar and Gluten-Containing Grains

These two foods alone are to blame for *so many* of the health challenges we're facing today. The staggering increase in our sugar and grains consumption over the past 60 years has corresponded with the rapid increase in inflammation, type 2 diabetes, obesity, hormonal issues, autoimmune conditions, cancer, heart disease, and more.

Fat has been blamed for all the problems that sugar has created, and sugar has almost been completely ignored. And grains? They're touted as the healthiest thing around by government health guidelines, the American Heart Association, Cancer Research UK, and Diabetes Australia to mention a few.

The U.K. government's Eatwell Guide guidelines for 2017 says that the majority of your daily diet should be bread, grains, pasta, and potatoes, and that toxic vegetable oils and margarine should be consumed daily. The U.S. guidelines are no better, recommending *11 servings* per day of grains, breads, and cereals. According to those bodies, you should have two slices of whole-grain toast *and* cereal *and* orange juice (a.k.a. a glass of sugar) at breakfast, a sandwich and fruit for lunch, crackers and fruit for a snack, and then spaghetti for dinner. The U.K. National Health Service recommends snacks[2] such as toasted cheese sandwiches, berry crumble, chocolate popcorn cakes, fish and chips, and pancakes with caramelized apple—and these are their suggestions for *children's snacks*.

These plans contain gluten and sugar at Every. Single. Meal. In fact, a day like that would have you consume over 400 percent more sugar than you should.

Whatever you've heard from your government, science says otherwise. Grains are not healthful! They increase inflammation,[8] lead to gut permeability, autoimmune conditions,[9] depression, and Alzheimer's disease.[10]

WHERE'S THE ACTUAL FOOD?

Every meal of processed, packaged, convenience fast food means another lost opportunity to eat fresh, healthful, nourishing, nutrient-dense foods. For many people, Big Food is all they eat.

As a dad, what really upsets me is how bad habits get passed down from generation to generation. Kids are even more susceptible to sweet Big Food in their bright, shiny packages, and they will always reach for that first. We need to teach our kids to reach for natural foods, but we also need to educate ourselves first. If things go the way they're going, one day, generations will grow up eating only grains, spuds, and corn. Eating five servings of fresh vegetables per day? For most, it's unthinkable, or a very rare event. According to the research I've done, five servings is the bare minimum we need. The barest of bare minimums. It should be 10 per day, and a colorful variety as well.

---

2   Seriously. Take a look at all their snack recipes: https://www.nhs.uk/change4life/recipes.

If we can simply up our fresh veggie consumption dramatically, we can reverse practically every health condition we face, even the most dangerous noncommunicable diseases. It doesn't need to be much more complex than this. Simply increasing your intake of fresh vegetables can make a huge difference in your body.

Your Health Is in Your Hands

Research has shown that many of the most widespread and threatening diseases—the ones most people think are due to bad luck, bad genes, or "just what happens when you get older"—are preventable through diet and lifestyle choices, according to research collected by the Centers for Disease Control and Prevention (CDC), Harvard University, and the Alzheimer's Association, to name a few. Some diseases preventable through diet are:

- Cancer: Up to 95 percent preventable through diet[11]
- Type 2 diabetes: 90 percent preventable through diet[12]
- Heart disease: 82 percent preventable through diet[13]
- Stroke: at least 80 percent preventable through diet[14]
- Alzheimer's: up to 99 percent preventable through diet[15]

Your health and your future are in your hands. No matter what your situation is right now, you can change and, quite rapidly, turn your health around and get to the energy, vitality, and body of your dreams. You just have to do things a little differently. And you'd be surprised at how little of a change can spark a cascade of incredible health and variety. You just need to know the things to focus on, the order in which to change things, and the levers to pull to make those changes as easy as possible.

Fortunately, you literally have the answer in your hands.

The Alkaline Reset Cleanse is the key to undoing years of damage, restoring balance to your body, fortifying and protecting it, and decreasing your risk of developing one of those awful, degenerative diseases. It gives your body a whole fresh, new start. I can't wait for you to begin *your* Alkaline Reset Cleanse and take action, so you can kick off your brand-new life of health, vigor, strength, energy, vitality, and ultimately, freedom.

But before you jump in, it's vital that you understand what's going on inside your body, and how the ARC is going to put all your imbalances back to rights.

CHAPTER 2

THE FIVE MASTER SYSTEMS

A healthy body is in balance; an unhealthy body is imbalanced. That makes intuitive sense to everyone who hears it, but what does it really mean?

When the body's many different systems are all humming along, doing what they should, you are in the desired state called *homeostasis*. There are many systems in the body, but nearly all of them are components of what I call the Five Master Systems (FMS). The FMS effectively control 95 percent of the bodily functions that are responsible for good health. They interact, work together, and cross over. Parts of one system are used by others. One system's mission impacts the others. They're all interconnected.

Their balance—both individually and interdependently—is the difference between abundant health for a lifetime or a rapid decline into sickness and disease. In this chapter, I'll introduce you to each system in the FMS, how it works and what can go wrong if it's not functioning properly. Don't worry. You won't need to break out your high school biology textbooks to keep up. But it is important for you to have a basic knowledge of your FMS so you can understand later how the Cleanse will reset, reboot, and rebalance each of these systems individually and in concert, to support them in everything they do.

THE FIVE MASTER SYSTEMS

The balance and health of these Five Master Systems is the difference between a life of energy and vitality and a life of daily struggle, fatigue, sickness, and disease.

1. Endocrine system
2. Digestive system
3. Immune system
4. Detoxification system
5. pH buffering system

The Endocrine System

Your endocrine system comprises hormone-producing organs and glands and the hormones themselves. Hormones are silent heroes, messenger chemicals that tell your body what to do. Without hormones, a woman's ovaries wouldn't know to release an egg each month. Your body wouldn't know to feel tired, or hungry (or full), or to run away from life-threatening situations. Right now, around 50 different hormones are calling the shots, controlling your biggest functions:

- Growth and development
- Metabolism
- Reproduction
- Body temperature
- Heart rate
- Blood pressure
- Appetite
- Body weight
- Response to stress and/or injury
- Digestion
- Mood

Each of your dozens of hormones are almost entirely regulated by a collection of important and super-sensitive glands and organs, including the hypothalamus, pineal, pituitary, thyroid, adrenals, parathyroid, thymus, pancreas, ovaries, and testes. Each gland and organ produces chemicals and sends those messengers back and forth with lots of cross talk, with one triggering the release of another, and some switching others off. If you saw it mapped, it would look like an insanely designed subway system with multiple layers and connections.

Much of this unbelievably complex system begins in the hypothalamus, a tiny area of the brain that largely controls the upper level of hormones (neurohormones, or, as I call them, "boss hormones"). The boss hormones, in turn, stimulate the stop and start of the lower level of hormones (the "worker hormones").

For example, corticotropin-releasing hormone, a boss, stimulates the adrenal glands to release corticosteroids, workers, to help regulate metabolism and immune response. Oxytocin stimulates the other hormones that control body temperature, sleep cycles, and the release of breast milk. Thyrotropin-releasing hormone stimulates the release of thyroid hormones that regulate metabolism, energy, and growth and development. And so on and so forth.

In an ideal world and a healthy body, the cascade of hormones flows perfectly. But we don't live in an ideal world, and most of us have to contend with hormonal imbalances that affect the other master systems as well. Because of its far-reaching nature, the endocrine system is a fantastic example of how one problem can lead to another. An imbalance might start in the endocrine system, but it will manifest in digestion issues, lackluster immune response, or high acidity. Or it might work the other way around, where digestive issues—and food choice—can trigger hormonal ones.

This Is Your Endocrine System on Grains

Specifically, I'm talking about gluten-containing grains like packaged bread, pasta, crackers, and chips—and even those supposedly healthy breakfast cereals. When you eat them, there is a *huge* spike in blood sugar. Just two slices of "healthy" whole-grain bread spikes your blood sugar even more than when you eat a chocolate bar.[1]

But how can that be?

Gluten-containing grains possess a specific carbohydrate called amylopectin A that drives blood sugar very high very quickly. That, in turn, causes the pancreas to release the hormone insulin. The higher the blood sugar, the more insulin that must be released to balance it.

If your blood sugar spikes repeatedly, your pancreas will *overproduce* insulin, which sets the wheels in motion to stockpile fat cells rapidly around your abdomen. The bigger your belly (i.e., the more visceral fat you carry), the poorer your response to insulin. When your body is slow to react to the overabundance of insulin, your pancreas will release more and more of it, which means more belly fat, which signals the release of more insulin, creating a vicious cycle. When things get really bad, visceral fat will accumulate, the flood of insulin will go out of control, and your body will become less sensitive to that hormone, making you "insulin resistant." And where do you end up? Being overweight, sick, and chronically exhausted.

Just to recap: Gluten-containing grains → high blood sugar → increased insulin production → increased insulin resistance → increased visceral fat → increased inflammatory signals → more insulin resistance → more overproduction of insulin → more visceral fat → more insulin production.

If this cycle continues unabated and unbalanced, too much insulin will stimulate overproduction of the adrenal hormone cortisol (a.k.a., the stress hormone), putting your body in fight-or-flight mode even when nothing is wrong. Elevated cortisol affects metabolism and sleep, creates inflammation, and lowers your immune response—and that's just *for starters*. Research has found it to be a precursor to *hundreds* of different conditions and illnesses, including the haywire productions of adrenaline, testosterone, and estrogen hormones. (Just as an aside, chronic elevated cortisol causes chronic acidosis, an imbalance in the pH buffering system, on the FMS,[2] another example of how it's all linked.)

At last count, Wednesday pasta night and a daily morning bagel have disrupted production of insulin, cortisol, adrenaline, testosterone, and estrogen, leading to visceral fat, autoimmune conditions and inflammation, fatigue, insomnia, and digestive issues, and the list goes on (and on). The irony is that, all along, we've been told that grains are healthy.

The endocrine system with its dozens of components and thousands of interconnections within itself and to the other master systems might seem so intricate that it would be impossible to balance at all, let alone *re*balance. But, you don't have to do anything to sort out the snarl of hormones in your body this minute. Right now, all you need is to appreciate how complicated it is and know that caring for all of your hormone-producing glands is not hard to do. You don't need a separate strategy or nutrient to heal each individual one. By following the ARC, you will be providing your body with all the tools it needs to balance and reset your entire hormone system and regain homeostasis, the perfect balance that leads to optimal health and energy for you and a much, much easier path to achieving your health goals. The solution to good health is actually very simple, no matter how complex the problem.

Endocrine System Disruptors

Some factors that jam your chemical messaging system include:

- Sugar
- Gluten-containing grains
- Meat
- Dairy
- Soda
- Dyes and additives in processed food
- Stress
- Toxins from pollution, cleaning, and personal products
- Poor-quality sleep
- Over-the-counter medicines

The Digestive System

Hippocrates, the father of medicine and creator of the Hippocratic oath ("first do no harm"), said, "All diseases begin in the gut."

He got that right 2,400 years ago!

Since Hippocrates's day, many other experts have agreed. They say the digestive system is your second brain and that your gut is the root of vibrant health. And it's 100 percent true. If your digestive health is out of balance, your general health will be off. Maybe you don't think of your gut as something you need to deal with given other issues you might have, like feeling tired all the time, or a skin condition, allergies, low libido, or foggy thinking.

But turn that thinking around. All of these symptoms are intrinsically linked to gut health. Gut problems are *not* just bowel-movement-based. Your gut is a vital part of the interwoven matrix that determines your health—in fact, it sits at the head of the table.

Your gut produces and manages several of the body's most important hormones, such as the fat-storage regulator leptin, the hunger hormone ghrelin, the insulin regulator enteroglucagon, and 22 other hormones that aid digestion, proliferate cells, regulate proteins, stimulate and release energy, and control appetite. Plus, your gut is home to the largest concentration of mood-altering neurotransmitters, including serotonin. If you have mood issues, they're not all in your head. Ninety percent of the body's serotonin is made in the digestive tract, *not* the brain.

Your gut houses 70 percent of the cells that make up your immune system. It literally removes waste from the body. It contains the fungus *Candida albicans*, which, when overgrown, is one of the body's largest contributors to systemic acidity.

The bottom line: Your gut *has to be* in balance for abundant health and energy. No matter what your goal—even if it's something totally unrelated to your gut, such as gaining muscle mass—balancing the digestive system is the key to success.

In Praise of the Small Intestine

The small intestine is such a spectacular organ!

You probably don't give it much thought—definitely not as much thought as I do—but take a minute to appreciate the biological marvel that it is.

The small intestine isn't that wide, but it is *long*—6.7 meters (22 feet) on average—a muscular tube that handles about 90 percent of the absorption and enzyme activity in the digestive process.

It's got three parts. The duodenum connects to the stomach and mixes food with enzymes, rebalances the pH, and breaks it down. Next, the jejunum's inner walls are folded over and over, increasing the surface area of the small intestine to a whopping 250 square meters—nearly 2,700 square feet—not so small after all! The folds are lined with microscopic fingerlike protrusions called *microvilli*. The microvilli reach out and grab (or absorb) nutrients to disseminate into the bloodstream and, from there, to every cell in the body. In part three, the ileum mops up whatever nutrients were not picked up in the jejunum and connects to the large intestine.

If you're not absorbing nutrients properly, your cells will go hungry, and any and every health challenge can get a lot worse.

The way we eat and live has a huge impact on these microvilli and their ability to do their work. If your small intestine is clogged with undigested matter, and the microvilli are blocked from absorbing nutrients, your cells go hungry. If your small intestine is overgrown with *Candida albicans*, a pervasive yeast and opportunistic fungus, it will smother your microvilli. And if you're eating a lot of grains—which actually break down and destroy microvilli—you know what I'm going to say. It's bad.

> For good health, you have to honor your incredible small intestine and allow it to do its job with the efficiency for which it was designed.

Let's talk about bacteria. Our gut is home to approximately 100,000,000,000,000 (100 trillion) microorganisms. Not a million, or a billion, or a trillion. A *hundred trillion*! Most people don't quite appreciate the scope of this. Right now, your gut contains more bacteria than the total sum of all the cells in your entire body. We are more bacteria than we are human!

(Cue the soundtrack for *Alien*.)

Gut flora is *supposed* to be there. Much of it is good for you and contributes to so many important processes in your body—immunity, metabolism regulation, hormone regulation, and so much more *on top of* digestion and gastrointestinal function. But some bacteria is bad for you, and causes problems. In a healthy gut environment, a huge variety of good bacteria can flourish, while bad bacteria is kept in check. Again, it's all about balance. Your gut flora's balance can easily be knocked off-kilter by the usual suspects of stress, excessive use of antibiotics and nonsteroidal anti-inflammatory drugs (NSAIDs), sugar, grains, toxic oils, and lack of dietary fiber from vegetables and fruits.

An imbalanced gut flora has recently been linked to conditions as far ranging as autism, depression, autoimmune conditions such as Hashimoto's disease, inflammatory bowel disease, and type 1 diabetes. More commonly, you might experience:

- Digestive issues such as constipation, chronic diarrhea, and too much or no intestinal gas
- Chronic bad breath
- Depression and anxiety issues
- Hormonal problems
- Menstrual complaints
- Prostate trouble
- High cholesterol
- Chronic vaginal infections
- Chronic bladder infections
- Osteoporosis
- Sarcopenia (loss of muscle tissue)

These are the issues that are directly related, and when you consider the indirect effects of imbalanced gut bacteria, you can see how it can impact practically every area of your health and every physiological goal.

The Immune System

Your immune system is an interactive network of organs, cells, and proteins that protect the body from viruses and bacteria or any foreign substances. It works to neutralize and remove these foreign invaders. It has the secondary role of recognizing when the body's own cells have changed due to an illness or fighting an illness.

Of the Five Master Systems you'll be getting back into balance on the ARC, the immune system is probably the most behind the scenes. When it's working properly, you don't even know it's quietly policing your body 24/7, going about its business like a team of highly trained security guards, constantly asking every inhaled, swallowed, or skin- and mucous-membrane-inhabiting organism, "Hey! Are you supposed to be here?"

Whether or not the foreign organisms cause disease is decided by the integrity of our immune system. For example, if it's working well, germs come in and are recognized as intruders, and the body expels them. But when you have an under- or overactive immune system, things can go wrong, really quickly, and this has an incredibly detrimental effect on the rest of the body, including the other four master systems.

If your immune system is *under*active, you're prone to suffering from colds and flu, of course. An underactive immune system can be serious, leading to severe infection, nervous system damage, cancer, and more.

If it's *over*active, autoimmune diseases such as Hashimoto's, rheumatoid arthritis, and chronic fatigue are more likely to kick in.

If the other master systems—especially the endocrine, digestive, and pH-buffering systems—are out of balance, overall internal inflammation (the leading cause of an overactive immune system) will increase. It can go the other way, too. A compromised immune system also *causes* inflammation that leads to adrenal fatigue, thyroid conditions, excess cortisol and insulin, difficulty processing acids, and the buildup of candida that unbalances digestion . . . and around we go.

It doesn't take a nutritionist, doctor, rocket scientist, or immunologist to tell you that eating badly, drinking excessively, not getting enough sleep or exercise, and living an unhealthy life will weaken your immunity. When you treat your body badly, you will always catch more colds and flus, break out, and feel run down. On the other hand, if you nourish and support your immune system with good foods, plenty of water, and lots of sleep and exercise, you stand a better chance of protecting yourself more effectively. As such, the ARC directly enhances your immune system and removes the danger factors that compromise it.

The Detoxification System

Detoxification is the work of a handful of main organs—the lungs, skin, digestive system, liver, and kidneys—but really, the liver and kidneys are the stars of the show. Together, they remove chemicals, used hormones, and dead cells from your blood, produce bile, and excrete wastes from muscle breakdown. They act like a giant filter for the whole body, working 24/7/365 for your entire life!

If these organs get bogged down and clogged, and their performance is impaired, toxins will build up in your body, with far-reaching ill effects on all the other major systems. While the liver can largely regenerate and rebuild itself within 30 days (though not after long-term abuse), the kidneys cannot. It's lucky you have a spare! The kidneys:

- Regulate proper fluid and electrolyte (mineral) balance in the body, which is vital for your cells to perform their functions and to control blood pressure.

- Support the acid-buffering system to regulate pH.

- Secrete a number of chemicals, which initiates the release of antidiuretic hormone and aldosterone (essential for sodium conversion).

- Filter blood at the volume of 40 fluid ounces per minute, a quarter of our total blood flow.

- Control excessive blood glucose and mineral imbalances.

- Excrete wastes from muscle metabolism and urea from protein breakdown.

- Flush out urinary irritants such as bacteria and excess fluid.

The kidneys are doing all this every minute of every day. Just like the liver, if the kidneys can't do their job properly—essentially, filtering waste and flushing it out in urine—unfiltered waste will recirculate in the blood and become stored in the body, leading to all sorts of nasty symptoms that impact the other master systems.

It has been proven that a high dietary-acid load (meat, sugar, grain, and dairy) can irreversibly damage the kidneys. Conversely, studies have found that an alkaline diet (greens, greens, greens) can *prevent* kidney damage and disease. In 2014, a researcher from Austria did a study that confirmed that an alkaline-rich diet of vegetables and alkaline fruits, supplementation with alkaline minerals such as sodium bicarbonate, and a reduction in acid-forming foods provided long-term benefits to the kidneys.[3] Other randomized studies found that adding alkalizing agents to one's diet might halt the decline of renal function of those with chronic kidney disease and have a long-term favorable effect.[4] What we eat matters. Our body's organs—specifically the organs in charge of keeping the others clean and healthy—suffer from a high-acid-load diet.

The other major detoxifying organ is the liver. It is a football-size, funny-shaped organ that is critical to your health, and it's one we just *have* to pay special attention to. If your liver is under stress and out of balance, you'll age twice as fast and you can forget *ever* getting in good shape, having energy, or being free from illness.

You absolutely must give your liver some love. It is so vital to protect because it:

- Cleans and filters the blood.

- Filters *everything* you consume.

- Removes toxins, dead and unhealthy cells, bacteria, and chemicals from the blood before they pass into the digestive tract, the skin, the respiratory system, and so on.

- Produces bile, which your body needs to digest and use dietary fats throughout the body.

- Creates proteins that repair and regenerate tissues and cells throughout the body.

- Synthesizes cholesterol, which is vital for basic functioning, and delivers it to your cells.

- Breaks down carbohydrates, proteins, and fats from the food you eat and turns them into useful compounds, thereby driving your metabolism.

- Processes fructose, and is the only organ that can do so (unlike glucose, which can be metabolized anywhere in the body).

- Stores energy in the form of mobilized-on-demand glycogen, a carbohydrate that fuels the body.

- Stores nutrients that, like glycogen, are ready to go as needed.

- Breaks down unrequited components in the body, including excess insulin (to a point), other hormones, and dead cells. In effect, it acts as a clearinghouse for the body.

The liver is constantly working its socks off and could use some support. We give it a break by not consuming toxins, such as drugs and alcohol, or high-acid-load foods and fruit. When the liver (or kidneys, or both) are stressed, your body's performance will be negatively affected in practically every area.

When people think of a cleanse or detox, they quite logically think about it in terms of removing toxins from the body. Most programs do this by simply removing the bad stuff from your diet—i.e., a "no coffee for a week" cleanse. But they don't go far enough. It's so important not only to remove the causes of toxicity, but to nourish, reset, and reboot the organs of detoxification. If you can do that, you take detoxing to a completely different level.

The pH-Buffering System

If you're already familiar with me and my work, or even just seeing the title of this book, I'm sure you are expecting me to talk about pH. Maintaining pH balance is absolutely essential, and this is the core of where the ARC was built.

Keeping your body within the incredibly important, tight pH range of your blood and other extracellular fluids is *the* holistic effort of your entire body. The magic number for blood is pH 7.365, right in the middle of the range from 0 (battery acid) to 14 (liquid drain cleaner). Except for the ever-so-slightly alkaline blood, the body is slightly acidic by design. Our daily processes—metabolism, hormone production, lymphatic functioning, what the body does to stay alive—create a small amount of acidity. This is why we have evolved with an acid-buffering system. This small buffer is pretty much exhausted every day by neutralizing the acids that our daily functioning creates.

When your body pH falls below target (*too* acidic), it's not pretty. Your kidneys will shut down, your heart will stop, and you will, quite quickly, die. Your body does *everything* and *anything* to prevent that from happening.

And yet, blood can dip slightly below the essential pH 7.365 without killing you. However, if it does this too often, you will contend with chronic diet-induced acidosis, a condition scientifically linked to most cancers, hypertension, cardiovascular disease, type 2 diabetes, irritable bowel syndrome, Crohn's disease, chronic fatigue syndrome, kidney disease, liver disease, brain conditions, depression, and more.

Diet-induced means the acidity comes from the standard modern diet full of sugar, gluten, fast food, takeout, refined foods, packaged foods, additives, chemicals, preservatives, colorings, flavorings, dairy, coffee, tea, soda, fruit juice, and alcohol. Throw in the stress of modern life, and your tiny buffering system is exhausted before you even get out of bed in the morning!

Instead of contributing to the body's acidity, why not give it foods that are alkaline forming? People started talking about just that circa 1999 to 2000, and there was plenty of excitement about alkaline diets. Of course, any new theory inspires as many critics as converts. Admittedly, there wasn't a lot of research back then to prove the theories, but there is now! Thousands of studies have proven that an alkaline-forming diet supports your body's pH and prevents the danger of diet-induced acidosis and the damage a dietary net acid load has on your body's internal environment, with particularly strong data about preventing cancer, osteoporosis, reflux, gout, inflammation, and digestion issues.[3]

When your digestive system isn't able to absorb and use nutrients (remember the impacted microvilli or overgrown candida?) your body is not getting alkaline goodies (calcium, magnesium, potassium, sodium, manganese, iron, zinc, antioxidants, and vitamins) to help buffer acidity.

When you suffer from diet-induced acidosis, the adrenals release excessive stress hormone cortisol, leading to inflammation, adrenal fatigue, and other nasties related to chronically elevated cortisol, including certain cancers and visceral fat.

Speaking of visceral fat, excess acidity encourages its generation, which then kicks off inflammatory signals. And guess what inflammation causes? Acidity. And acidity causes inflammation.

The solution to this merry-go-round from hell is an alkaline diet.

---

3   There are references to a lot of these research studies throughout this book. I'm big on the research, but to get an even more comprehensive discussion of the science and research behind the alkaline diet, go to www.rossbridgeford.com/arc.

Just to be absolutely clear (this point is a source of confusion for many): *You're not trying to raise your pH on an alkaline diet.* That would be physically impossible (see above, regarding your body doing *anything* and *everything* it can to keep your blood at pH 7.365). But you *can* support your body in its effort to maintain the right pH. You *can* make it easier. By living and eating alkaline, we relieve the body of this regulatory need, and thus the body thrives. Of course, it helps (and is surely no coincidence) that alkaline foods are nutrient-dense, live, fresh, have a high water content, and are packed with vitamins, minerals, phytonutrients, and antioxidants.

Your body thrives in balance. By supporting it to do the *only* thing it needs to do—maintain homeostasis, keeping that balance—you can experience incredible health and longevity. The point of the ARC is to fuel your body and give it the tools it needs to effortlessly maintain that blood pH of 7.365.

In chapters coming up soon, I'm going to list acid-forming and alkaline-forming foods, and explain how something that seems acidic (like a lemon) is actually an alkaline food, and how some acid (like the stuff in your stomach) is good for you.

For now, I want to make sure that you understand the goal of an alkaline diet, regardless of the specifics, so you'll succeed at it. Rest assured, I will guide you the week before and the week during the Cleanse—you don't have to do anything but follow it. And when you go back into the wild on your own after that, you will have the science behind it and clear guidelines to easily continue on your own.

The alkaline diet—the way I teach it and what it is intended to be—is a *very* simple approach to health. The only goal of it is to give your body the foods that allow it to effortlessly maintain the delicate pH balance in your blood and other extracellular fluids at the slightly alkaline pH 7.365.

All the research that I've studied and gathered on my own in the past 15 years indicates that practically all preventable diseases are caused by three things:

1. Excess acidity

2. Excess inflammation

3. Oxidative stress

When the body is under constant attack from acid-forming foods, drinks, and other lifestyle choices (such as stress and lack of sleep), it can survive. But the body being forced to fight for survival is what kills you. It is the stress and pressure from constantly buffering that causes long-term damage and disease.

By cleansing and balancing the FMS, with a particular emphasis on the pH-buffering system, you will keep acidity, inflammation, and oxidative stress in check.

In the next chapter, I'm going to explain what each of the three horsemen of your body's apocalypse are, and the specific damage they can cause.

Worst-Case Scenario

I want to talk about a condition called leaky gut (and, yes, it's just as bad as it sounds). It's the end result of the perfect storm when one system failure sets off the next, resulting in body breakdown.

And it all starts with eating gluten-containing grains.

For starters, as soon as these grains reach the intestines, the gluten is broken down into two proteins, gliadin and glutenin, by an enzyme called transglutaminase (tTG). As proteins make their way through your digestive tract, your gut identifies gliadin as a dangerous substance and produces antibodies to attack it.

The problem is, the antibodies produced by the tTG to attack gliadin *also* destroy and erode the digestive system superstars and nutrient-absorbing microvilli. An *overactive* immune response results in damaged microvilli, which might already be matted down in undigested matter. Either way, they can't do their job, and you don't wind up digesting any of the nutrients you consume.

First symptom: all day—day in, day out—fatigue, no matter what you eat. You could be eating superhealthy, but because your digestive system is not able to extract any of the goodness and nourishment from the food, you'll be lacking nutrients and therefore will have extremely low energy and a considerably imbalanced digestive system.

To make this worse, grains also contain the *anti-nutrients* phytic acid and lectins. Phylates are mineral blockers that prevent absorption of the critical alkaline minerals calcium, magnesium, iron, copper, and zinc. Lectins are proteins that simply cannot be digested. When they pass through your gut undigested, they further damage microvilli, cause inflammation, and knock your overstimulated immune system further off balance. Increased inflammation means cortisol overproduction and higher acidity. Meanwhile, clogged intestines prevent the absorption of water and other liquids, minerals, and electrolytes, so your detoxification system is compromised, too.

Are you keeping track? The endocrine, digestive, immune, detox, and buffering systems are all out of whack. In very little time, after repeated exposure to grains and these lectins, chronic inflammation loosens the junctions between cells in the gut wall. Holes will appear in the intestines that allow toxins to pass through. This process is helped along by another gluten protein called zonulin, which independently contributes to loosening those junctions.

Not good.

The border wall has been breached. Intestinal permeability (a.k.a. leaky gut) means that toxins and intruders can get *into* your gut, and also that undigested food—literal waste—can get *out* to your bloodstream, along with the millions of random viruses, bacteria, and indigestible molecules like dust and other stuff you swallow every day that should go out the other end. Your immune system will go into overdrive to deal with all this muck, putting you at high risk for a plethora of autoimmune conditions, including chronic fatigue, adrenal fatigue, thyroid disorders, Hashimoto's, and rheumatoid arthritis. Also throw in insulin resistance and type 2 diabetes.

Leaky gut is arguably one of the most common and potent factors in practically every health challenge we're facing right now. It's truly a disease of civilization that is caused by poor diet and is the end result of one bad thing inevitably leading to another.

CHAPTER 3

YOUR BODY'S NUMBER-ONE GOAL

We know our standard American diet (or what I call the "standard *modern* diet" because not only America eats this way) is responsible for thousands of conditions and sicknesses, such as cancer, heart disease, liver disease, osteoporosis, fibromyalgia, and acid reflux.

We also know that these diseases are caused by and contribute to imbalances in the Five Master Systems. Imbalance is at the root of practically every health challenge. While *your* personal goal for your body might be to look fabulous or to feel full of energy, *your body* has one simple goal: to keep you alive. To do that, it has to maintain balance. Balance equals life.

Your body will drop *everything* and do whatever it takes to prevent blood pH imbalance from happening, and the death it can quickly cause. Yet there are severe consequences from the drastic measures the body takes to *recover* from imbalance.

Just because the body *can* regulate these balances does not mean we should force it to do so. When you are out of balance, your body goes into "red alert" mode, putting damaging stress on your entire system. The effort the body goes through to correct the imbalance is like the cleanup after a hurricane. You survived the storm but are left with the wreckage and no electricity or clean water. Your body's journey from a diet-induced state of acidity *back* to its normal baseline can result in insulin resistance,[1] type 2 diabetes,[2] hypertension,[3] chronic kidney disease,[4] muscle loss,[5] cancer,[6] osteoporosis,[7] and so much more.

The collateral damage of red-alert mode is called "toxic load." For example, when an imbalanced endocrine system overproduces cortisol, the body has to balance the chronically elevated levels. In this process, it creates a by-product of excessive acid. That toxic acid load then winds up creating imbalances in the pH-buffering and digestive systems. Fighting to balance one system puts undue stress on the body and leads to *more* conditions and toxicity that allow *more* disease to emerge.

The body's primary goal is to keep you alive. If that means creating longer-term problems, that's what it's going to do, even if the results are devastating. It's only a matter of time before you pay the price for existing in red alert, a lot sooner than most people think. Some imbalances that cause long-term catastrophic consequences include:

- Diet-induced acidosis

- Poor gut bacteria ratios

- Elevated hormone production—in particular, the overproduction of insulin and cortisol

- Elevated white and red blood cell production

- Overactive immune activity

- Production of free radicals

- Overproduction of digestive system acids

- Over- or underproduction of enzymes

Just one imbalance—the good-to-bad gut bacteria ratio—can ultimately cause such conditions as constipation, chronic diarrhea, chronic bad breath, hormonal problems, PMS, prostate issues, breast enlargement in men, a rampant candida infection, chronic respiratory problems, high cholesterol levels, neurological problems, and osteoporosis.

Chronically elevated cortisol can trickle down to cancer[8] and heart disease.[9]

A chronically overactive immune response to excessive inflammation can cause autoimmune conditions such as rheumatoid arthritis and lupus.

The body's overcompensation to try to manage the balance of hydrochloric acid to sodium bicarbonate production during digestion causes acid reflux.

Osteoporosis is often a result of the body being unable to buffer excess acidity from the standard modern diet.[10]

Gout is a result of the liver failing to properly metabolize fructose and an overproduction of uric acid, a toxic load by-product from an imbalance in the detoxification system.

These examples are just a handful of what can happen when your body is constantly in red alert and fighting back to balance. It's sort of like an action movie, when the heroes go from one disaster to the next. They survive, but they leave nothing but destruction in their wake.

The way people eat, drink, and live in our modern society forces their bodies to struggle from the moment they wake up until the moment they go to sleep. They might not realize it (yet), but they are fighting a losing battle all day, every day, just to try to maintain the critical balances that keep them alive. And the more sugar, grains, soda, bread, pasta, and fast and processed foods they consume, the more out of balance they are, and the deeper the hole (dug with a fork) becomes.

If you bombard your cells with junk and deprive them of nutrients, it is only a matter of time before chronic imbalance leads to something serious. It might start small. Maybe you feel more tired than you'd like. Maybe you get aches and pains from time to time. After a while, your complaint might become something upsetting and uncomfortable, but not life-threatening, such as irritable bowel syndrome or acid reflux. And then, in a little while, if the imbalance is not attended to, that annoying IBS develops into leaky gut—and now the poop, literally, really starts to spread. A leaky gut almost always turns into an autoimmune condition like Hashimoto's disease, knocking your thyroid out of whack, which can then target adrenals like a smart bomb. Bring on the weight gain, anxiety, fatigue, mental fog, and poor sleep *on top of* the IBS, acid reflux, aches, and pains. Now life is a constant struggle. Cancer probably comes next, and it could cut your life short.

All because of imbalance.

Five Master Systems Imbalance Consequences

An imbalance within each of the Five Master Systems can rapidly result in long-term problems, including the following.

Endocrine system: thyroiditis, adrenal fatigue, type 2 diabetes, osteoporosis, reproductive issues, metabolism disorders, and some cancers.

Digestive system: acid reflux, IBS, Crohn's, diverticulitis, gallstones, and peptic ulcers.

Immune system: rheumatoid arthritis, Hashimoto's disease, lupus, multiple sclerosis, and thrombocytopenia.

Detoxification system: liver disease, kidney disease, fatty liver, gout, and nervous system damage.

pH-buffering system: take your pick, since diet-induced acidosis and inflammation can negatively impact practically every process, area, and organ in the body.

Most people who eat the standard modern diet may not realize that it lights a fuse inside their bodies. The cumulative imbalance, if not addressed, can explode into fatigue, foggy thinking, anxiety, weight gain, an inability to lose weight, aches, pains, being *under*weight and unable to gain weight, reflux, IBS, gout, arthritis, and osteoporosis. If *any* of these symptoms sound familiar, they are clear signs that your body is imbalanced.

You might be surviving, but just barely.

YOUR BODY NEEDS YOUR HELP

The food, drink, and lifestyle choices you make *today* will directly affect the delicate balance of these intricate systems in your body *immediately*, whether positively or negatively.

You can make lasting, permanent positive change if you improve your diet today. However, if you've been eating the standard modern diet for years—and have been yo-yo dieting to take off excess weight—the battle happening inside your body could be even more challenging.

According to a 2017 study by researchers in England, the body will buffer as much diet-induced acidity as it possibly can, and whatever it can't neutralize is stored in the body.[11] Over time, the toxic by-products build up in tissues. Bone and muscle are the first things to deteriorate under the burden of stored acids. When the body has an overload of stored uric acid, the extremities swell, which can be a symptom of gout.

One "bad diet" storage problem is all too familiar to most of us. Excess production of insulin—largely from consuming gluten and sugar—causes the rapid formation of visceral fat cells, which are difficult to lose on any "diet." Once the body stores something, it's not too quick to let it go, even if it's harmful to your health. A rapid overgrowth of candida in the digestive system—the by-product of digesting sugars, yeasts, gluten, and processed foods—obviously interferes with digestion and you'd think the body would do whatever it could to get rid of it. In fact, it tries to, with an immune system response that causes inflammation and more acidity, and pretty soon, the buildup of candida and undigested matter clog the small intestine, preventing nutrient absorption and possibly causing leaky gut.

There are *hundreds* of examples of how stored toxic loads force the body into a "state of emergency" each time it has to rebalance. And when we keep forcing this rebalancing on our body, things get chronically out of control, because each of these problem areas *further* contributes to an ongoing chronic imbalance.

Your first clue that your system is imbalanced might be as innocuous as a skin condition, bad breath, or poor energy. As the imbalance progresses, the second clue might be something debilitating but not life-threatening, such as acid reflux, IBS, gout, or thyroiditis. Your last clue would be a life-threatening degenerative disease like cancer or heart disease.

It can get so bad that even if you started eating well right now, your body would have to stay in red-alert mode to deal with the sheer amount of toxic buildup in the body. The imbalance from these stored toxins in and of themselves have to be addressed before the effects of the toxins can be healed.

In other words, you have to cleanse out the toxin buildup first in order to give your body a fresh start.

After I explain all this, clients often ask me, "How do I know if I'm just imbalanced or if I'm dealing with years of stored-up toxic load?"

The reality is, it doesn't matter. Regardless of whichever you think it might be, you need to rebalance and reset. Everybody is different, with many variables such as how much sugar and gluten you eat, your genetic makeup, your exposure to external toxins (chemicals, pollutants, and transferable germs/diseases), your medication use, and your environment. But regardless of the toxicity in your individual body, you need to rid yourself of toxic load *and* assist your body with getting back in balance and maintaining it, without killing yourself in the process. To rebalance effortlessly—the not-so-secret secret to vibrant health—you have to cleanse out the overages and inflammation, giving your body every tool it needs to repair, rebuild, and thrive.

CLEANING OUT TOXICITY TO REBOOT THE SYSTEM

If you've been living in a state of imbalance for years, are already experiencing symptoms, or are currently dealing with a health challenge, you need to take massive positive action. And, I'm sorry to say, a salad here or there won't cut it. Nor will a glass of lemon water in the morning. While delicious, it isn't going to fix you.

You need a reboot.

You need to break the vicious cycle by hitting the reset button and cleansing your master systems that have been so imbalanced for so long, repairing the organs and systems that are responsible for maintaining balance.

The ARC is going to help you to do this powerfully and rapidly with an abundance of nourishment, undoing years of clogging and imbalance and giving your body a fresh start with full function and strength.

You will be working *with* your body to support it and help yourself heal. You and your body are a team. When you work together, you can work wonders. So join forces! Give your body, your*self,* a wholehearted "Thank you!" for getting you this far, and show your gratitude by giving it the nourishment it needs to say, "You're welcome!" If you do that, your body will repay you tenfold.

CHAPTER 4

THE TOP THREE IMBALANCERS

System imbalance is primarily caused by unhealthy food and drink choices, and then by long-term toxic load buildup that keeps your body in red-alert mode—in other words, actively fighting its way back to homeostasis.

In the previous chapter, I touched on exactly what toxic load is. Now I want to do a deep dive into the three main imbalancers that disrupt your Five Master Systems; they are the root cause of practically every sickness and disease we know of. The ARC was designed to address and correct these imbalances. But before we get into *how* the ARC rids you of these toxins, it is essential that you understand what they are and what causes them.

THE TOP THREE IMBALANCERS

To win the fight for a life of energy and good health, you have to know your enemy. In this case, there are three:

1. Acidity
2. Inflammation
3. Oxidative Stress

1. Acidity

The regulation of your pH after consuming acid-forming foods is a very complex process that starts in the digestive system, where the pH potential of food has a direct, instant impact on the ratio of hydrochloric acid and sodium bicarbonate produced in the stomach during the first stage of digestion. If you bombard your body with acid-forming foods (sugar, grains, meat, dairy, alcohol, chemicals, hydrogenated fats, and trans fats), you enter a state known by the medical community as diet-induced acidosis, low-grade acidosis, or chronic metabolic acidosis.

When you consistently put your body into diet-induced acidosis (the term I prefer), things start to break very quickly, and in a multitude of ways.

In the past 80-plus years, medical science has proven **a clear link between an acidic diet and the incidence of cancer.** In one recent study, researchers from the Harvard School of Public Health and the University of Southern California analyzed data from 41,731 women between the ages of 35 and 74, and found that diet-induced acidosis was a significant risk factor for invasive breast cancer.[1]

In a recent Japanese study,[2] the researchers analyzed the health records of 31,590 adults who underwent a health screening between January 2001 and December 2010 and found that those with the lowest (acidic) urinary pH had a far higher incidence of cancer and cardiovascular mortality than those with the highest (alkaline) urinary pH.

Thousands of studies have shown the protective effect against cancer of consuming a diet rich in alkaline vegetables and fruits. In April 2017, Chinese researchers conducted a meta-analysis that covered more than 10,000 individuals, and showed that the higher the participant's vegetable consumption, the lower their risk of renal cell carcinoma.[3]

The Alkaline Cancer Conversation

You might have heard people say that cancer cannot exist in an alkaline environment. That theory came from famous German physiologist Otto Warburg in his 1931 Nobel Prize–winning study. At first glance, you'd think *Wow!* But when you dig a little deeper . . .

This is something I call a "dotted line theory." It sounds right on paper, but can't actually be substantiated when it comes to our diet and the foods we eat. Our friend Otto Warburg wasn't studying the link between acid and disease to show the benefits of the alkaline diet. He was researching it to expand our understanding of cancer. His research is right—cancer can't live in an alkaline environment—but this is only relevant *in vitro*, i.e., in a test tube or outside the body.

We can't re-create the same condition in the body through diet. The body regulates the cells and organs at the exact pH they need to be—the stomach pH, 2 to 4.5; the duodenum and pancreas, pH 7 to 7.5; the small intestine, 7.4; the large intestine, pH 5.5 to 7; lymphatic fluid, 7 to 7.5; gallbladder, 6.8 to 7.5; and so on. By eating alkaline, the body won't then go alkaline everywhere! If it did, you'd die with a condition called *metabolic alkalosis*.

While it is true that an acidic environment increases the risk of cancer occurring and that eating alkaline is designed to remove that risk, I want to set the record straight about these myths and how all this plays into the ARC.

You are not trying to re-create Warburg's *in vitro* environment.

Eating alkaline won't make your whole body "turn alkaline" and kill the cancer cells.

When you "eat alkaline," you are giving your body an abundance of nutrients to do the best it can to fight disease. An alkaline diet *will* support the body in maintaining homeostasis, and within that balance, it will increase its ability to prevent cancer.[4]

Simply put, the alkaline diet is an incredibly powerful *preventive* measure.

If you have cancer, it will give your body the perfect environment to rebalance and heal. But it is misleading to say, "Cancer can't live in an alkaline environment, so make your body alkaline." It's not possible to "make your body alkaline," and saying so opens up the good work of alkaline-eating proponents for undue criticism.

Acidosis doesn't stop with cancer. According to the CDC, one in four deaths in the U.S. are due to cardiovascular disease (CVD). One of the main causes of CVD is diet-induced acidosis. In a 2017 study published by the American Society for Nutrition, researchers investigated more than 90,000 individuals and found that those with a higher dietary net acid load had a higher risk of total mortality, particularly from CVD. This confirmed the findings of Korean researchers who, in 2015, looked at the health screenings of 31,590 adults and found a correlation between acidosis and a significant increase in the risk of CVD.[5]

What about weight gain and type 2 diabetes? Is diet-induced acidosis to blame there, too?

A diet high in acid-forming foods (sugar, chips, soda, pizza, ice cream) and low in alkaline-forming foods (leafy greens and vegetables) will likely lead to weight gain, but not for the reasons you might think. It's an oversimplification to say it's just a matter of calories in versus calories out. Science has proven that type of model to be a very poor predictor of long-term weight loss and gain.

The relative speed of weight (fat) gain or loss and its longevity (how hard it is to lose it), comes down to several related factors, including your hormones, gut bacteria, and inflammation, with diet-induced acidosis at the core of all of them.

For one thing, acidosis completely messes with two hormones that are vital for weight loss—leptin and adiponectin. Leptin is responsible for sending the "stop eating" message to the brain. If leptin is suppressed, you are more likely to feel hungry *all the time*. According to the findings of a 2003 Swiss study,[6] acidosis significantly decreased leptin levels. In other words, if you're acidic, you're always going to be hungry. If you're always hungry, you're going to reach for the fastest, easiest food—most likely unhealthy options—throughout the day.

Just as important is adiponectin, the hormone that tells your body to burn fat for fuel. In a 2010 study,[7] Thai researchers simulated metabolic acidosis in participants over seven days, and found that within that time period, the levels of circulating adiponectin in the body were significantly decreased. In effect, the subjects were burning less fat for fuel after only a week of high acid food intake.

Rounding out the hormonal nightmare, diet-induced acidosis causes chronically elevated cortisol, which can trigger inflammation, fatigue the adrenals, and imbalance gut bacteria, all of which are heavily responsible for fat-cell formation, weight gain, and an inability to lose weight. This potent cocktail for fat increase makes it incredibly difficult to decrease over the long term.

Even more dangerous than excess weight is type 2 diabetes, a chronic illness that can lead to strokes, kidney diseases, CVD, and blindness. Acidosis strikes again by increasing cortisol levels, which has been proven to promote insulin resistance, meaning an increased risk of a huge number of metabolic diseases.[8]

Due to the detrimental effect of diet-induced acidosis on thyroid function,[9] an acidic diet can have serious effects on our body's ability to regulate other cancer-fighting hormones such as insulin-like growth factor (IGF), which is essential in protecting against prostate, colorectal, and breast cancer. This deleterious effect on the thyroid—the increased production of cortisol and the promotion of insulin resistance—also contributes to the increased risk of adrenal fatigue.

2. Inflammation

Inflammation is alarmingly prevalent in our society. Practically everyone is carrying inflammation in their body to some degree simply because of the volume of pro-inflammatory foods eaten day in, day out, though many are also living under high levels of cortisol-inducing stress.

Unless your diet has been very clean and alkaline for many years while you have had incredibly low stress levels, you are likely carrying inflammation and experiencing its far-reaching, and often quite devastating, effects. If left unchecked, chronic inflammation can cause autoimmune diseases, leaky gut, digestive issues, thyroid and adrenal issues, arthritis, inflammatory bowel conditions, chronic fatigue, cancer, heart disease, diabetes, kidney disease, liver conditions, and, most definitely, cognitive issues (from depression to dementia).

Chronic inflammation has long been linked to cardiovascular diseases; in recent years, the research has been coming to light to prove it. A 2016 study at the University of California, Los Angeles, found a correlation between higher inflammatory biomarkers and an increased prevalence of coronary artery disease (CAD).[10] If your heart is clogged with plaque, it's also inflamed, and due to the inflammation, you'll wind up with more plaque.

Next, diabetes. Inflammation comes into play with faulty insulin signaling, too. According to a 2009 Austrian study,[11] inflammatory markers, known as cytokines, can interfere with insulin signaling, resulting in increased insulin resistance and spiked blood sugar. The spikes trigger white blood cells to attack, and inflammation continues. In addition to increasing the risk for diabetes, insulin resistance can make you gain weight.

One thing a lot of people don't realize is that mood disorders are often the consequence of physical problems, not necessarily or completely due to psychological ones. According to a 2015 study by Canada's Centre for Addiction and Mental Health, depressed people had 30 percent more brain inflammation than those who were not depressed. Inflammation can also increase your risk for age-related cognitive decline and dementia, as researchers from the University of Pittsburgh concluded in their 2013 study.[12] The research on inflammation and brain conditions has uncovered some remarkable links between diet and neurological disorders such as depression and Alzheimer's. The bottom line is that inflammation affects the brain in a major way.

Prevention of cancer through lifestyle factors is an exciting new avenue of study. Organizations such as Cancer Research UK have reported that when the body becomes aware of a fledgling tumor, the immune system kicks in, and the area is flooded with oxygen-carrying blood cells and nutrients—the inflammation process—but instead of killing the tumor, it actually helps it grow. If that inflammation response can be stopped, scientists are hoping that the tumor can be starved.

3. Oxidative Stress

Before I can get into how diet and lifestyle cause oxidative stress, let's first define some terms.

Oxidation: Basically, oxidation is what happens when something comes into contact with oxygen. Examples found outside the body include rust and an apple turning brown after it is left on the counter. When oxidation happens inside the body, a similar thing happens. The cells start to degenerate. This might be confusing, because we breathe oxygen, and, through metabolism, change air into energy. Without oxygen, our cells would die. The simplest explanation I can give you about the seeming contradiction is that to live is also to die a little every day. In effect, oxidation *is* aging.

Free radicals: The process of changing air into energy creates the by-products we know as free radicals. We create them all day, every day, just by our body doing its basic functioning. Some free radicals attack infections and are important players in your immune system. But other free radicals roam your bloodstream looking for unpaired electrons to gang up with. Ordinarily, your body can balance your free-radical levels. But if you have too many of those scavenger free-radical atoms, they cause oxidative stress inside the body. Think of them as rust particles that, if abundant and clumped together, will corrode your insides.

It's all about balance yet again. If you have too few free radicals, your immune system, digestive system, and detoxification systems are in trouble. But if you have too many, they'll destroy cells, alter your DNA, and age you way faster than you can believe.

This phenomenon is called rapid premature aging (RPA) and, like acidosis and inflammation, it's caused by the standard modern diet and poor lifestyle choices (not enough sleep, scant exercise, stress, toxins, repeated use of prescription and OTC drugs). We are producing far more free radicals than we can handle. The body is overrun and can't dispose of them all.

Does this sound similar?

Remember how the body creates acidity through normal bodily functioning, so humans evolved an acid-buffering system to deal with it? But through diet and lifestyle, our bodies are exposed to tons more than we can handle and get sick as the result. It's the same process with free radicals. Our bodies are built to deal with a trickle, but we're giving them an avalanche. The result: oxidative stress, which damages DNA, weakens cellular membranes, and clogs your blood vessels with fat—which, in turn, kicks off rapid premature aging.

If rapid aging doesn't kill you fast enough, perhaps some of the other conditions associated with oxidative stress will, such as certain cancers, atherosclerosis, Parkinson's disease, immune system disorders, rapid weight gain, liver damage, heart disease, asthma, and diabetes.

A Bonus *Fourth* Imbalancer

In covering the sources of imbalance, the picture would not be complete without including stress.

I don't mean internal stress on cells (like oxidative stress). I mean the day in, day out feeling of being constantly under the gun. This one doesn't have anything to do with food or drink, but it is about lifestyle and how you prioritize your life.

Study after study has shown how elevated cortisol (the fight-or-flight hormone released when you feel stressed out) has a deeply profound impact on your health. As we have already discussed, cortisol is a precursor of so many conditions and health challenges, including cancer and heart disease.

The bottom line is that worry, concern, anxiety, and all the other negative emotions related to stress cause a spike in cortisol, which is *always* profoundly unbalancing. Not only does it tax the adrenals, hypothalamus, pituitary gland, and other organs and glands within your endocrine system, it also increases acidity,[13] inflammation,[14] and insulin resistance,[15] which leads to diabetes.

If there is anything I've learned in life, it's that emotional stress can take you down a very slippery slope with your health. You need to put things in place to help manage it. You cannot prevent stressful events from occurring, but you can control your reaction to those events.

For me, the single-biggest tool I found for staying positive and handling stressful situations as they pop up has been the Headspace meditation app. I have absolutely no affiliation with Headspace, but it was life-changing for me, so I wanted to bring it to your attention. It *is* meditation, and some people react negatively to that. But check it out, just once; it's free. Headspace makes it so easy. Just 10 minutes a day can be a game-changer. Within three days, it changed my whole outlook. I learned how to observe my negative thoughts with a degree of detachment instead of allowing them to take over, for example.

Whether it's exercise, yoga, sex, singing, dancing, therapy, meditation, cats, cat videos, or goats in pajamas videos, you need to find what works for you to relax and quiet the sirens in your head. The Alkaline Reset Cleanse will *absolutely* help clear your mind and lift your outlook. You will feel empowered instead of helpless about your health. When coupled with a regular mindfulness practice, the results can be exponential.

Now We Know the Nature of the Beast

Now that you get that your body *has* to maintain balance at all costs, you can turn that knowledge into a golden opportunity. Understanding what your body needs makes it easier to understand what *you* need to do to help it: Choose alkaline foods and drinks, and de-stress your life.

Think about your last 48 hours. What did you eat? How well did you sleep? Did you laugh or exercise? Did you contribute to *balance* or *imbalance*?

Has your diet increased or decreased acidity, inflammation, or oxidative stress?

Have you been working with your body or against it?

What you eat and do every day—for good or ill—has a lasting, profound effect. The next positive step in your journey toward balance and good health is learning about the *antidote* to imbalance in order for your body to thrive.

I hope that you are excited to join me on the health-promoting road now, leaving baggage and bad habits behind.

Or, in other words, moving onward to Chapter 5 . . .

CHAPTER 5

BACK IN BALANCE WITH THE TRIPLE A METHOD

Acidity, inflammation, and oxidative stress are the primary sources of imbalance. In other words, they are the root cause of any health challenge you're facing right now.

So it's not too surprising that the solution to practically every sickness and disease is their opposite: alkalinity, anti-inflammation, and antioxidation.

By making dietary and lifestyle changes, you can swing the pendulum of your health in the right direction—and keep it there. You'll notice that each antidote starts with the letter *A*, which is why I call my plan the **Triple A Method**. The beauty of it is that nearly all the recommended foods in the plan tick *all three* boxes. It is rare to find a food that is *only* alkaline without providing anti-inflammatory and/or antioxidant benefits as well. Similarly, there is rarely a food that is *just* anti-inflammatory or *just* antioxidant-rich. An approved food might result in more of one benefit or the other, but it always provides a well-rounded effect on the body.

When you think of only consuming foods and drinks that are Triple A Method approved, you have a powerful, guiding principle to make the right choices. Nearly all the time, those choices will be intuitive. With just a little guidance (which, of course, I'll provide), you'll be able to switch, effortlessly, toward alkaline, anti-inflammatory, and antioxidant-rich goodies. The research so clearly points to the foods that prevent and cure so many of the health challenges we face today, and they are delicious, fresh, packed with flavor, and come in abundant variety!

During the seven days of the ARC, I'm going to give you very specific recipes and shopping lists. But when you finish the Cleanse and go back to your day-to-day life, you'll have a very good idea of what foods to choose. You don't need to be 100 percent perfect—even trying to be perfect is a recipe for disaster. Just shoot for eating Triple A friendly foods most of the time. Look, I'm a realist. I know people are going to have a burger, pizza, and ice cream every now and then. When you do, just make sure you have some countermeasure foods alongside.

If you can dramatically reduce acidity, oxidative-stress, and inflammation (as much as humanly possible—it's not possible to *completely* eradicate them), you will look and feel like a million dollars in very little time.

Now, let's go through each of the As:

Alkalinity

If you want vibrant health, you have to "go alkaline." The core of the Alkaline Reset Cleanse is built around this tenet (first clue: the name!). But what on earth does "go alkaline" mean?

As a quick science refresher, pH is the measure of acidity or alkalinity ranging on a scale from 0 (the most acidic) to 14 (the most basic/alkaline), with pH 7 right in the middle, as neutral.

Different areas of your body require a different pH. Saliva ranges between 6.5 and 7.5. The upper stomach has a range of 1.5 to 4; the duodenum ranges from 7 to 8.5. And the small and large intestine go from 4 to 7, depending on where they are in the digestive process.

The one constant pH is your blood. It *has* to stay slightly alkaline at 7.365. As you now know, the body will do whatever it takes to maintain that pH. If it dips, your body goes into a state of emergency, and if pH doesn't get back to level, your organs will start to shut down until you die. Think of your blood pH as the first domino. If you knock it over, it will knock over every other bodily function one by one.

The logarithmic scale that measures pH in food and drink is complicated, but bear with me. Anything with a pH of 6 (white rice, for example) is 10 times more acidic than a substance with a pH of 7 (such as oats). A substance with a pH of 5 (condiments such as ketchup or fruit jam) is 100 (10 squared, or 10 x

10) times more acidic than the pH 7 foods. A pH of 4 is 1,000 (100 squared, or 100 x 100) times more acidic than a pH of 7, and so on. Each one pH point is a square of the one before.

Cola has a pH of 3. Every sip does damage (let alone drinking many cans per day).

What you eat and drink absolutely has a *huge* impact on the blood pH.[1] A diet that weighs more heavily in acid-forming foods and drinks is effectively a prescription for sickness and disease. The prescription for health? Naturally, it's to eat an alkaline diet. The way I teach it, that means the *majority* of your food and drink has a supportive, nutrient-dense and alkaline-forming effect in the body and limits those that have an acid-forming effect. It is not about being 100 percent perfectly alkaline. Aim for 80 percent and you'll do yourself a world of good.

Acid/Alkaline Food Chart and More Downloadable Resources

I have included an "At-a-Glance" reference chart of common acid- and alkaline-forming foods on page TK, but to download a full chart with 400-plus foods ranked from Strong Acid to Neutral to Strong Alkaline, go to your Alkaline Reset Cleanse Resources page at https://www.rossbridgeford.com/arc.

You'll find everything you need to put the ARC into practice, including all of your meal plans, recipes, shopping lists, and day-by-day action plans—plus bonus resources like my "How to Go Alkaline" guides and more.

Humans evolved to eat alkaline.[2] All the foods on my approved list existed and were eaten by our preagricultural ancestors. Think of big, vibrant, colorful plates of real, whole, nourishing, natural foods that are stuffed with vitamins, antioxidants, nutrients, protein, and healthy fats. I'm talking about vegetables like spinach, kale, beetroot, broccoli, and bell pepper; plenty of healing fats and oils from coconut, avocado, almonds, cashews, and seeds; proteins from quinoa, oats, lentils, and kidney beans. It's all rooted in the JERF philosophy of "Just Eat Real Foods."

Alkaline foods in, acidic foods out. Stay away from sugar, gluten-containing grains, processed foods, fast foods, cakes, biscuits, microwave meals, processed meats, and sugary drinks and snacks. You know the stuff. That's why going alkaline is so intuitive. Eat fresh veggies, drink lots of water, go outside and exercise, and don't sit around indoors eating rubbish. That's pretty much it in a nutshell. Your grandmother has said as much your whole life.

You can't argue with nature, common sense, or Grandma. It is no coincidence that naturally alkaline-forming foods are the ones *anyone* would consider healthy and that acid-forming foods are those everyone *knows* are unhealthy. A 2014 study[3] identified the most "powerhouse foods," assessing their micronutrient content (vitamins, minerals, and antioxidants). Of the top 41, 38 were alkaline forming. The top 15 were all leafy greens.

It isn't even about being vegan, vegetarian, paleo, or ketogenic (although the alkaline approach is aligned with paleo and keto). The way I teach my alkaline approach is designed to be fun, easy, and achievable, so you can eat meat and have treats, and you can still go out to dinner with your family or friends and have the occasional blowout. You never have to be perfect. You are simply working toward alkaline majority and making veggies, healthy fats, and plant proteins the stars of the show 80 percent of the time.

There's more detail to it than that, and I will cover everything you need to know within the ARC program. But I wanted to explain it to you first in super-simple terms because that is exactly what it is. Simple. And easy to get on board.

The Alkaline Reset Cleanse is my recommended first step, without question. Ninety-five percent of the people I work with have some degree of acidic buildup, candida overgrowth, inflammation, and oxidative stress in their body. You need a thorough cleanse to start fresh for rapid healing. Even if your diet is pretty solid already, the ARC can clear loads of stored toxins, bad bacteria, acids, and digestive clogging you had no idea your body was clinging to. After all, the by-products of acidosis, inflammation, and oxidative stress are made by your body every day. It's a good idea to clear them out with a full cleanse to reboot your systems. Who doesn't like a clean slate?

During the seven days of the Alkaline Reset Cleanse, you will need to be as perfect as you can possibly be. Look, it's only a week. You can do anything for just seven days. And then once the Cleanse is over, add more of the good stuff, and steer away from the bad stuff meal by meal, day by day, and so on, until the transformation is complete and alkaline foods are the mainstay of your diet. You'll feel so energized and healthy, you won't want to go back.

Going Alkaline in a Nutshell

- Focus your diet around fresh foods, vegetables, greens, and salads
- Eat an abundance of healthy fats
- Stay well hydrated and exercise
- Avoid sugar, gluten-producing grains, trans fats, and processed foods

That's it! Really!

There are literally thousands upon thousands of published papers that support the benefits of alkaline foods, and a 2012 University of Alberta, Canada, study summed it up best, concluding that alkaline diets "benefit bone health, reduce muscle wasting, as well as mitigate other chronic diseases such as hypertension and strokes." The lead researcher, Gerry K. Schwalfenberg, went on to say, "An alkaline diet may improve many outcomes from cardiovascular health to memory and cognition. . . . it would be prudent to consider an alkaline diet to reduce morbidity and mortality of chronic disease that are plaguing our aging population."[4]

It's all about supporting your body. Remember, the single goal of your body is to maintain balance, and my alkaline diet gives the body every tool it needs to thrive *and effortlessly maintain this balance*. It's not about changing your pH. Rather, it is about consuming an abundance of the foods that will support your body in its task of balancing your pH as effortlessly as possible.

Some people believe that just because the body has a pH buffering system and *can* maintain the blood's slightly alkaline pH that you don't need to worry about it. In other words, go ahead and eat deep-fried Mars bars for breakfast, lunch, and dinner, washed down with a six-pack of Coke and turn your nose up at greens.

I cannot understand this. Why force your body into a constant struggle? Having to neutralize diet-induced acidity is hugely stressful and damaging to your kidneys, liver, thyroid, adrenals, digestive system (especially the stomach and pancreas), bones, brain, lymphatic system, and lungs. By focusing your diet on alkaline-forming foods, and limiting those acid-forming foods, you will be giving your body a *huge* helping hand. Plus, you'll have energy to burn, a clear head, and a calm mind.

Alkaline Superstars

Spinach

All leafy greens should be eaten in abundance, but spinach is my absolute favorite because it's easy to buy and easy to use in recipes and salads—and it's delicious. Baby spinach and fully grown spinach are nutritional powerhouses and are incredibly alkaline. As with all green foods, spinach is rich in chlorophyll, the stuff in plants that makes them green.

Q: What is the most essential substance that your body uses to build and transport red blood cells, which is absolutely vital to blood volume and health?

A: Hemoglobin. It's a protein that's in charge of transporting oxygen in your blood; in fact, your blood is approximately 75 percent hemoglobin.

Q: What promotes and supports your body's hemoglobin?

A: Chlorophyll. Its molecular structure is almost identical to hemoglobin except for the center atom. In hemoglobin, it's iron; in chlorophyll, it's magnesium (an essential alkaline mineral). When ingested, chlorophyll (in liquid form, such as in juices, smoothies, and soups), helps to rebuild and replenish your red blood cells, boosting your energy and increasing your well-being almost instantly. I know this sounds a bit like the ancient food myth, like eating brains makes you smarter. But eating and drinking chlorophyll *does* increase the quality and quantity of your red blood cells.

Whenever you eat or drink something green, you are alkalizing your body and building your blood. A handful of spinach is in nearly every recipe in this book. Along with potent chlorophyll, it's sky-high in vitamins A, B complex, C, E, K, manganese, folate, magnesium, iron, calcium, potassium, and dietary fiber. I doubt there is a more all-around healthy food on earth, and I highly encourage you to eat spinach throughout the day, every day.

Kale

Long known in my circles as one of the *most* alkaline foods, kale is another leafy-green beauty that is heralded for its cancer-fighting, cholesterol-lowering, antioxidant-rich, detoxifying goodness. It's less popular than spinach, only because it has a history of being cooked poorly, like cabbage. But when it's properly prepared, it is absolutely delicious.

Like spinach, kale is massively high in vitamins A and K, and, being a leafy green, it has a huge chlorophyll content. The reason it is *such* a powerful weapon against cancer? It contains at least four glucosinolates, compounds in pungent foods (such as cabbage, mustard, and horseradish) that fight disease.

As soon as you eat and digest kale, these compounds are easily converted by the body into cancer-fighting warriors. Also, kale—especially steamed—is quite amazing for lowering cholesterol.

Cucumber

The beauty of cucumber is its phenomenal 95 percent water content. You won't find that anywhere else. Owing to that, cukes provide an alkalizing, tasty, nutritious base for practically every ARC soup, smoothie, and juice.

Along with being an incredibly hydrating food to consume, it also contains a superb amount of antioxidants, including the super-important lignans. These highly beneficial polyphenols are usually associated with cruciferous vegetables, but their content in cucumbers is widely acknowledged, too. The big three lignans in cukes are lariciresinol, pinoresinol, and secoisolariciresinol, all of which have been proven to reduce the risk of cardiovascular disease and cancer of the breast, uterus, ovaries, and prostate.

In terms of the nutrient recommended dietary allowance (RDA) per serving, cucumbers contain fair amounts of vitamins K and C, some A and B, and loads of alkaline minerals, including calcium, iron, phosphorus, potassium, magnesium, selenium, copper, manganese, iron, and zinc.

Broccoli

Broccoli is a must. If you are serious about living with health, energy, and vitality, you simply have to eat broccoli, if not on a daily basis, then at least four times per week.

Broccoli has been proven, many times over, to inhibit cancers and support the digestive, cardiovascular, and detoxification systems, as well as improve skin, boost metabolism and the immune system, serve as an anti-inflammatory, and provide ample antioxidants.

One of broccoli's powerful compounds, and the reason it is included in the ARC in such abundance, is sulforaphane. Sulforaphane is the closest thing to a panacea we've got. It's highly alkaline, powerfully antioxidant, and strongly anti-inflammatory, which makes it a Triple A triple threat. You'll find this compound in most cruciferous vegetables (cauliflower, cabbage, brussels sprouts), but its highest concentration is in broccoli. Please, please, please eat lots and lots of it—steamed, roasted, or raw. Put it in salads, juices, smoothies, and soups. I sound like a broccoli addict! I am! I don't let a meal go by without thinking, *How can I get some broccoli in here?*

Avocado

I'm even more addicted to avocados! I eat a *lot* of them, at least one per day in every salad, smoothie, or soup, sometimes more.

I know some people give the avocado a bad rep because 85 percent of its calories come from fats. But that makes no sense. You need fats to live, and avocados provide an excellent source of them that will never make you gain weight. If anything, due to the high content of oleic acid (an omega-9 fat that's very similar to olive oil), it can *lower* total cholesterol, raise your high-density lipoproteins (HDLs, a.k.a. "good cholesterol") and lower low-density lipoproteins (LDLs, a.k.a. "bad cholesterol"). Oleic acid slows the development of heart disease and promotes the production of antioxidants. These beneficial omega oils also help speed metabolism, which will help you *lose* weight!

Avocados are packed with a wide range of other nutrients that have anti-inflammatory, heart, cardiovascular, anticancer, and blood sugar benefits, as well as the key antioxidants alpha-carotene, beta-carotene, lutein, and selenium.

Plus, halved with a squirt of lemon and sea salt? What is more delicious?

Celery

Celery, like cucumber, is alkaline and has a high water content, making it a perfect base for juices and soups (not smoothies, though, because you have to juice it first, and then you have twice as much cleanup).

Celery contains two lesser-known beneficial nutrients: phthalide, a compound that lowers cholesterol, and coumarin, a cancer inhibitor. It's also rich in vitamin C, an antioxidant that supports the immune system and cardiovascular health and reduces inflammation, which is very helpful for fighting arthritis, osteoporosis, and asthma.

If you are on a weight-loss journey, you'll also be happy to hear that this alkaline staple contains plenty of potassium and sodium, diuretic minerals that help rid the body of excess fluids.

Watercress

Watercress tops the list of powerhouse foods. It contains no less than 15 essential nutrients. It has more iron than spinach, more calcium than milk, and more vitamin C than oranges.

Similar to the other greens listed here, watercress is rich in chlorophyll, making it a great alkaline blood builder. It's also high in antioxidants such as gluconasturtiin, the highly anticarcinogenic compound that gives it a peppery flavor.

Watercress is abundant in calcium, manganese, and magnesium, as well as vitamins A, C, and K, making it fantastic for your bone health.

I absolutely love watercress in salads, soups, smoothies, and juices, and if you haven't fallen in love with it yet, I really recommend that you do!

ANTI-INFLAMMATION

Similar to acidity, the toxic by-products of inflammation can hang around and get stuck in the body, leading to problems of their own, like candida overgrowth, visceral fat-cell formation, insulin resistance and autoimmune conditions, among others. Fortunately, the cure is located at the farmers market.

Prior to the last 10 years or so, inflammation was seen more as a *reaction* to other conditions in the body. When scientists realized inflammation was the *cause* of problems, they began to investigate the link to diet, and all the info about food's anti-inflammatory capacity rapidly emerged. At the time of this writing, there were more than 11,000 studies about the thunderous impact of one food as an anti-inflammatory wonder: turmeric. Thousands more studies have heralded the anti-inflammatory powers of ginger, garlic, omega-3 fatty acids, coconut oil, broccoli, beetroot, and avocado.

Of course, inflammation is a natural response in the body. When you cut yourself or get an infection, your immune response kicks in, rushing blood to the area, causing a normal important response called "acute inflammation." Symptoms of inflammation might be redness, swelling, heat, joint pain, or muscle pain. It's happening to me right now. Yesterday I fell over a suitcase (I know) and my knee is hot, red, bruised, and swollen. Acute inflammation . . . happy days!

However, when the immune response gets locked in the "on" position and won't switch off, *chronic* inflammation occurs: Inflammation deep in your tissues refuses to recede appropriately, and your organs become gummed up with excess swelling, hormones, and enzymes. Your body believes it's fighting an imminent threat where there is none.

And here's the thing: Chronic inflammation is caused by diet and lifestyle.

The usual suspects are to blame. Not to worry! Triple A foods will take care of it, no problem. On the ARC, you will be getting a *lot* of the most powerfully anti-inflammatory foods, while all pro-inflammatory foods will be eliminated.

The result is a huge relief for your body—the ability to heal, removing inflammation and repairing the damage it's caused.

By rebalancing away from acidity and inflammation, you will feel an incredible difference. But there is the third and last Triple A healing source to discuss—*antioxidants!*

Anti-Inflammatory Superstars

Turmeric

Turmeric, a root you probably don't think about much, has powerful anti-inflammatory, antitumor, and antioxidant properties. It contains a pigment called curcumin that gives it a yellow-orange color, and is the active ingredient behind many of its health benefits. One Italian study[5] had 50 osteoarthritis patients take 200 milligrams of curcumin per day. After three months, the subjects experienced reduced pain and increased mobility, whereas the control group, which received no curcumin, experienced no significant improvements. Other research also found that a turmeric extract composed of curcuminoids (plant-based nutrients that contain powerful antioxidant properties) blocked inflammatory pathways, effectively preventing the launch of a protein that triggers swelling and pain.

Clinical studies have also found that curcumin has very powerful antioxidant effects, enabling it to neutralize free radicals and dramatically reduce joint inflammation and pain. It's definitely worth including in your daily diet—but don't get it on your clothes unless you wear a lot of orange. I learned that lesson the hard way on dozens of occasions!

Ginger

Ginger contains ultra-potent anti-inflammation compounds called gingerols. Gingerols have been proven to provide pain relief from inflammatory conditions like osteoarthritis or rheumatoid arthritis. In clinical studies with patients who responded to conventional drugs and those who didn't, physicians found that 75 percent of arthritis patients and 100 percent of patients with muscular discomfort experienced relief of pain and/or swelling if they took gingerols daily.[6] Ginger is delicious, easily used in cooking, juices, and smoothies, and really adds spice to your life.

Garlic

Delicious, smelly, and darn good for you, garlic has huge anti-inflammatory properties that have been linked to cardiovascular health, prevention of obesity, and in helping and preventing arthritis. Two additional compounds in garlic—vinyldithin and thiacremonone—are found to inhibit the activity of inflammatory messenger molecules while also providing an antioxidative stress benefit. The most researched compound in garlic, allicin, has been linked to many anti-inflammatory benefits, making garlic a food that should definitely be eaten multiple times daily.

Beets

As with many other high-antioxidant foods (yep, they show up on that list, too), beets have been shown to have fantastic anti-inflammatory benefits. The phytonutrients betanin, isobetanin, and vulgaxanthin found in them have been the subject of huge amounts of research with regard to heart health (a symptom of chronic inflammation). Alongside the anti-inflammatory benefits that betanin has, it is also proven to have antifungal properties and aids in detoxification.

Asparagus

Asparagus is a super-anti-inflammatory because of its unique combination of nutrients, including asparanin A, sarsasapogenin, protodioscin, diosgenin, quercetin, rutin, kaempferol, and isorhamnetin. You don't need to be able to pronounce those, nor do you need to remember them. Just know that asparagus has more anti-inflammation compounds than any other food!

Plus, asparagus contains antioxidant stars vitamins C and E, beta-carotene, and the minerals zinc, manganese, and selenium. What a winner!

Flaxseed

Omega 3 is crucially important to fight inflammation. The primary omega-3 fatty acid in flaxseeds—alpha-linolenic acid or ALA—is fantastic for the cardiovascular system in and of itself. It acts as a building block for other molecules that help prevent excessive inflammation and protects the blood vessels from inflammatory damage. But the antioxidant and anti-inflammation benefits of flaxseed don't stop there. Research has found that omega-3 intake prevents inflammation-based conditions including high cholesterol, high blood pressure, heart disease, diabetes, rheumatoid arthritis, osteoporosis, depression, inflammatory bowel disease, and asthma. Grind it up and sprinkle it on anything and everything you eat!

Coconut Oil

Coconut oil, a healthy saturated fat, is a known anti-inflammatory, analgesic, and fever reducer that you will be consuming in abundance on the ARC. If you are still worried about saturated fats being bad for your arteries, please relax. This is an old, debunked, outdated theory that has been dispelled by hundreds of research studies. I know, it's scary to think that the advice you've been told for decades was wrong all along. But we have irrefutable evidence to prove coconut oil and other saturated fats are healthy.

It's an anti-inflammatory.[7]

It ignites metabolism.

It balances hormones.

Its lactic acid is antimicrobial.

It fights candida[8] and is an especially powerful enemy of inflammatory arthritic pain.[9]

You should feel great about consuming coconut—its oil, milk, and cream—before, during, and after your Cleanse. It's very safe to cook with (although on the ARC, you won't be doing much "cooking"), making it the best oil for frying, baking, and anything else. (Other oils—including olive—become toxic when exposed to heat, light, and air.) Oh, yeah, it tastes *delicious*, too, giving your soups and smoothies an exotic flavor you will adore.

ANTIOXIDANTS

Of the three Triple A sources, antioxidants are probably the most familiar to you. We've been hearing about the benefit of antioxidants for years. But when you ask someone what they are, or what they do, the response might be a blank face.

Antioxidants are the direct remedy to oxidative stress. If you recall from the previous chapter, oxidative stress is literally the process of your cells rusting from too many free radicals circulating in the body. Remember, we need *some* free radicals; balance here is key, as always. The standard modern diet and lifestyle kick free-radical production into orbit and out of balance.

I mentioned that free radicals are atoms in search of a lost electron, and their rampaging quest through the body is what harms it. Antioxidants simply donate the missing electron back to the free radical and neutralize the danger. It's as simple as that. By consuming an abundance and variety of antioxidants—as you will throughout the ARC—you give your body the weapons it needs to fight oxidative stress, but also to balance the levels of free radicals circulating throughout your system, allowing your body to repair the damage.

There are dozens of different antioxidants, and each have their own strengths and particular benefits, ranging from eye health to cancer prevention. But rather than focusing in on the specific benefits of specific antioxidants, it's more important to aim for a wide variety of food sources to give you an exceptional blend of antioxidant benefits.

In the ARC, throughout the before, during, and after stages, you will be getting an incredible variety and volume of antioxidants—some you have already heard of (like vitamin C, vitamin E, and beta-carotene), and some you might not have heard of, such as:

- **Lutein and zeaxanthin.** These two carotenoids (colorful pigments) are found in kale, spinach, bell pepper, and broccoli, and are known to support eye health and prevent macular degeneration.

- **Quercetin.** This polyphenol is found in spinach, lettuce, tomatoes, bell peppers, asparagus, and buckwheat, and is known to fight inflammation, protect against heart disease, nourish the skin, and more.

- **Pinoresinol, lariciresinol,** and **secoisolariciresinol.** Lignans (natural chemicals from plants) are found in cucumbers, cabbage, kale, sesame seeds, and olive oil, and have been proven to protect against hormone-related cancers.

- **Catechin.** A flavonoid found in green tea and cocoa that helps prevent heart disease.

- **Isorhamnetin.** A flavonoid found in red and yellow onions that can suppress skin disorders.

- **Apigenin.** A flavonoid found in parsley and celery shown to be anticarcinogenic.

A full list would go on forever. Besides, you don't really need to know their names. Just attempt to include a huge volume of colorful veggies, seeds, and healthy oils in your diet to boost your antioxidants. I want you to think beyond the mainstream obvious ones, like blueberries and green tea (which aren't, actually, the richest sources), and turn toward veggie sources like kale, bell pepper, beets, carrots, asparagus, and red onion, and healthy oils, as well as nuts and seeds.

On the ARC, you will be flooding your system with many powerful, plentiful antioxidants to work their healing magic. Like the other two As in the Triple A Method, antioxidant-rich foods are also alkaline and anti-inflammatory, too. Nearly every food on your ARC shopping list will have fantastic crossover benefits!

Antioxidant Superstars

Bell Peppers

The humble bell pepper—red, green, yellow, or orange—is sweet, crunchy, and refreshingly delicious. You can use it in almost any meal—raw, grilled, fried, roasted—and it is always a winner. If you're missing sweetness when you first start to "go alkaline," then bell pepper can bridge the gap.

Inside every red bell pepper are dozens of antioxidants, including vitamins A, E, and more C than an orange, plus flavonoids, carotenoids, and hydroxycinnamic acids. The bell pepper actually contains more than 30 different members of the carotenoid (the red, yellow, and orange pigments) family. The only other food that comes close to that is the tomato. Just a sampling of what bell peppers can do for you: decrease the risk of cardiovascular disease, type 2 diabetes, macular degeneration, cancer, and inflammation. And if that's not enough for you, they crunch! Better than chips!

Carrots

Carrots are an abundant source of biotin, vitamin A, C, and K, molybdenum, and potassium, as well as carotenoids (alpha- and beta-carotene and lutein), hydroxycinnamic acids, and anthocyanins (trust me, they're all really good for you). Carrots' potent combo of antioxidants promote eye health,[10] as well as cardiovascular, bone, and liver health, and ward off certain cancers, too. You'll get plenty of carrots during the Cleanse in juices, smoothies, and soups, giving you a little sweetness without the life-clogging fructose found in fruits.

Alfalfa Sprouts

Alfalfa sprouts are uniquely skilled at lowering the production of free radicals *and* reducing free-radical-caused cell death and DNA damage. The high quantities of isoflavones and other phytoestrogens (plant-based sources of estrogen) in alfalfa have been proven to have strong anticancer properties, especially with breast and other hormone-based cancers.

Like many of the foods in this chapter, alfalfa is high in vitamin K, manganese, and magnesium, making it a strong bone builder. Alfalfa sprouts are such an easy addition to any meal, just by throwing a handful into a blender, juice, or soup. You can easily grow them at home using a sprouter or purchase fresh from the store. As with all sprouts, they are such a tiny powerhouse food, you don't need to use a lot to get a ton of benefits.

Brussels Sprouts

Similar to asparagus, brussels sprouts are rich in kaempferol, an antioxidant linked to fighting cancer[11] and inflammation. One recent study discovered that when participants ate about two cups of brussels sprouts daily, the damage to their cells from oxidative stress decreased by 28 percent.[12] Other research concluded that brussels sprouts might be stronger cancer fighters than broccoli.[13] Their sulforaphane (a compound also found in broccoli and cabbage) makes them heart protective, too. Perhaps most impressive, brussels sprouts contain the relatively rare sulfur-containing compound called D3T, a powerful detoxifier that supports your body's detoxification phase one (breaking down toxins into particles) and two (eliminating toxins). Both are important. Without an effective phase one of detox, phase two doesn't work. And without phase two, the toxins remain in your body!

By consuming plenty of brussels sprouts, you're not only supporting your body's efforts to uproot and break down the toxins stored in your system, but you're supporting its effort to remove them, too, both of which are critical during the ARC.

A DIET THAT REPAIRS, REBOOTS, AND RESETS YOUR ENTIRE BODY, INSIDE AND OUT

One hundred percent of the foods you will eat in abundance during the Alkaline Reset Cleanse are Triple A approved. Since you'll be consuming absolutely *zero* acidic, inflammatory, or oxidative-stress-causing foods, you will be locked into healing and balancing mode for the entire seven days.

Acidity, inflammation, and oxidative stress—the Destroyers—are closely related, intrinsically linked, and, when combined, are more powerful than the sum of their parts. The damage of acidity, combined with oxidative stress and inflammation, is exponential.

But the power of a diet rich in alkalinity, antioxidants, and anti-inflammatory foods is also exponential, and even more powerful. Your body wants to be healthy. It wants to be in balance. All you have to do is help it do what it wants to do by giving it Triple A foods.

So let's get started! In Part II, you'll learn exactly what the Cleanse is, and how you'll go about doing it.

Gail's Story

After 44 years working shift work and as a paramedic, it would be fair to say it had taken its toll on my body. I was constantly tired, feeling sluggish, never sleeping well. I wouldn't say I was depressed, but every day I felt flat. I hated the way my body had become. I had gained weight and I knew it was not going in the right direction. Even though I don't drink a lot, I had been diagnosed with fatty liver and I could see things were going in the wrong direction.

I needed something to change, and the push came in a very unexpected place—on a cruise ship! I went to a talk about the alkaline diet and a woman I sat next to in the audience told me about Ross, and about how she'd lost nine kilograms (nearly 20 pounds) following Ross's alkaline plan, and I thought, *Why not . . .*

I joined Ross's Cleanse, and it was amazing. Everything he said just made so much sense to me. It felt natural, and Ross made it all so easy.

I must admit, before the Cleanse started, I did wonder, *Am I going to be able to do this? Will I be able to stick to it?* But it was so easy. I was never hungry; I never had any cravings—not even for sugar, which had always been my downfall. But with Ross, the food is divine, it's not hard, it's really tasty, it's fresh, and even my husband, who was always a meat and two veg kind of guy, is in the kitchen now, cooking the meals for me, and he's loving it too.

My life now, after the Cleanse, is unrecognizable. And all I did was follow it! It was so simple! I lost 30 centimeters [nearly 12 inches] of fat from my body—5 centimeters [2 inches] from my waist and thighs. I am getting so many compliments. My skin is great, I'm getting into clothes I hadn't been able to wear for years, and it is just fantastic.

I had a DEXA (bone-density) scan before I started, and I was 42 percent body fat, which was frightening. But now I'm already down to 31 percent and I couldn't be happier.

My future has just opened up so much. I'll be around for my kids and my grandkids for a lot longer now. All I wanted as I got older was to be able to stay independent and to see my grandkids grow up, and that is what I have to look forward to now.

This has opened up a whole new world for me to have fun and be vibrant. Thank you, thank you, thank you so much for giving me this. It's a gift I can never repay; all I can do is spread the word. It's been fabulous for me—a massive big thank you and a big kiss!

Gail is a client of the full online Alkaline Reset Cleanse program (joined September 2017).

PART II

RESET
YOUR
HEALTH

CHAPTER 6

THE FIVE PILLARS OF THE ALKALINE RESET CLEANSE

All you have to do is start with the Alkaline Reset Cleanse. It takes you from where you are now to where you want to be, with absolute simplicity and ease. Putting rocket fuel into a beat-up old car isn't going to turn it into a rocket. For those who have spent years yo-yoing or eating the standard modern diet, you have to rebalance and unclog the Five Master Systems and eat Triple A foods in abundance to reboot your body into a state where it can run optimally. The ARC is the reboot. Once you've completed it, you'll notice the benefits extend (and often get bigger) for weeks and months afterward. You'll reexperience a whole new level of health and energy you last felt as a kid.

The benefits of the ARC go beyond the body. Vibrant health and energy positively impact every area of your life and make everything a little bit easier. Tens of thousands of my clients have reported improved mood, outlook, time management, relationships, careers, and finances. But, as I've heard over and over, achieving any career or financial goal isn't nearly as joyful and satisfying if you have to sacrifice your health to do it. With the ARC, you sacrifice nothing except the things that are making you suffer body and mind. It's all about abundance and gain. You will take control of your health, and your other goals will feel attainable. Imagine what you'd be able to do with 10 times the energy you have now, while thinking clearly and staying focused for hours longer and waking up earlier. It's like giving yourself several extra *active, energized, optimal* hours each day.

As you go through this life-changing process, please keep the five pillars of the Cleanse, the focus of this chapter, in mind. But the one über-pillar is that the ARC is going to be a pleasure. While getting a whole new lease on life, you're going to feel excited and happy. I've designed the ARC to be easy and enjoyable. If the ARC weren't simple and fun, people wouldn't do it! Or they'd start, hate it, and stop, and I wouldn't blame them. Misery is not sustainable, and quitting is *the last thing* I'd want to see happen.

As anyone can tell you, the most effective health plan is the one you can stick with. And that's precisely why the ARC is so effective. My 92 percent completion rate is the stat I care most about, more than pounds lost and conditions remedied. I'm confident that you will love the process and grow more enthusiastic as you go along.

Now, on to the five pillars . . .

Pillar #1: Nourish, Not Punish

Some believe that the goal of a cleanse or detox program is to starve out the toxins by starving yourself. You have to endure exhaustion, constant hunger, mood swings, and dreaded detox symptoms for seven days with the hope that feeling awful will all be worth it in the end. The most widely held theory is that you have to restrict what goes into the body to give it a "break" and force it into detoxing, so you consume practically nothing (think consuming only lemon water and maple syrup for days) and hate every minute of it.

I fundamentally disagree with this approach.

Rather than being miserable and "toughing it out," I prefer to question whether any positive results are short or long term, as well as causation- or correlation-based. In other words, did the cleanse succeed because of the lemon water and maple syrup, or was it the fact that they cut all the acidic, inflammatory, and oxidative foods and drinks like caffeine, alcohol, trans fats, sugar, gluten, and dairy? My guess would be that, in a lot of cases, the latter is true. (I'm always open to being proven wrong. Fifteen years ago, I used to think that whole grains like spelt and couscous were okay. Nowadays, I won't touch the stuff and highly recommend you don't either. Science moves on; new things are discovered and proven—or disproven.)

The ARC is not a detox plan. If you are looking for pain and suffering, you have come to the wrong place.

My plan is not grueling or punishing or something you have to "get through." It's not about restriction; it's about abundance. It's not a fast; it's about nourishing yourself all day long.

Willpower? Not required. The seven days of your Cleanse will be joyous, energizing, and satisfying. You'll feel full yet light. My overall philosophy of health is to give the body what it needs to thrive. On my Cleanse, you will be asking the body to do a *ton* of work to completely clear out and reboot, so *why* would you restrict the nutrients you need to do that? My approach is to give you *more* awesome nutrients, not less!

Your body knows how to do its job. It's the most effective self-repairing, rebuilding, and regenerating system in the world. It just needs to be unlocked. Flooding it with antioxidants, vitamins, minerals, anti-inflammatories, and alkaline goodies is the key. I have seen such dramatic results with the ARC; I am absolutely convinced that this is the most effective way to look after and fuel your body.

The ARC is a long-term plan. It's a seven-day process solely devoted to getting you a clean slate, which you can then build on with even more enthusiasm. After that first week, you will feel amazing—primed, reset, and restored. Your system will be back at its best, everything clean and clear, functioning perfectly and efficiently, and internally in the best shape it's been for decades.

I think of the last day of the Cleanse as a new Day Zero, the first of the rest of your life of abundant health and energy, with perfectly restored and balanced Five Master Systems. It's not about a quickie last-minute extreme diet to get you into a smaller-size dress for a wedding or any other kind of short-term goal that perpetuates the yo-yo weight loss/gain eternal cycle in the first place.

No, no, no. The ARC's objective is to get you back to optimal functioning, and then to enjoy the increasingly enhanced benefits for months, if not years, *afterward.*

It's Not a Diet, It's a Lifestyle

One of the most powerful—and most important—steps in making this approach "stick" for life is called "Crowd Out the Bad Training." I really want you to put these concepts into practice and make this happen. In your ARC Resources, I have included one of the key video lessons from the full online Alkaline Reset

Cleanse program for you so we can go deep on this. I also include the full work-book and step-by-step Action Plan on how to put this into practice, so don't miss them! Head to www.rossbridgeford.com/arc to access this, plus all of your other ARC guides and resources (including your printable recipe books, meal plans, and shopping lists).

Once your body is reset and rebalanced, continued healthy living will have a bigger impact than when you were putting healthy foods into a clogged-up body. Your body can now efficiently and effortlessly use the nutrients you provide. It doesn't have to use all its energy just to keep you alive, neutralize acids and toxins, and battle free radicals and bad gut bacteria. Your body is humming along, using almost no energy now, and so you feel like a million dollars.

The ARC kicks off the beginning of a new lifestyle. You will want to keep the effects going because they feel that good. But you don't have to be perfect! You'll be in such fantastic shape internally; you can have treats, nights out with friends, and barbecues. With powerful, healthy, reset master systems, your body can cope with occasional acid-forming foods and drinks, and recover more quickly from them.

Unclog for Keeps

If your digestive system is clogged, you could eat all the veggies in the world and take the highest-grade green powders, and your body *still* wouldn't be able to assimilate and disseminate (i.e., take in and spread about) those nutrients.

Typically, if you have a clogged digestive system, you will only absorb a small percentage of the nutrients in the best salad ever compared to someone who has a perfectly functioning, clear digestive system. On the ARC, you will unclog your intestines by . . .

1. **Waking up sluggish microvilli.** When you eat junk food, these hair-like sponges along the walls of the small intestine get matted down. On the Cleanse, you will clear the sludge and the microvilli will stand at attention, ready and able to soak up nutrients.

2. **Clearing candida.** When in proper balance, *Candida albicans*, a parasitic fungal yeast, can actually support the body by aiding in nutrient absorption and digestion. But, on the standard modern diet, fed by sugar and spurred on by antibiotics use, candida flourishes wildly. The truly gross and insidious nature of candida: It feeds on its own waste.

Overgrowth leads to more growth, and it can be difficult to get levels back under control. Medication is not a long-term option. Candida is actually a part of your normal flora, and you want a little of it. Rather than kill it with medication and sheer force, the smarter strategy is to starve it to cull it back. This is exactly what the ARC will do with balance-restoring coconut oil, greens, anti-inflammatory roots, and alkaline-forming foods, and, of course, by eliminating sugar, gluten, grains, and processed foods. If you've ever had any candida issues (or if you have them now; many people do without realizing), you're going to *love* the results of the ARC.

Once you unclog your gut, you will start to absorb nutrients at a much higher percentage. Your entire body will be replenished, and you will feel radiant and alive. You have to be patient, though. It takes a week or so to clear the gut. But once it's functioning again, *BANG*, it will start absorbing nutrients like crazy. This is exactly what I mean when I say the benefits *really* kick in after the Cleanse, because that's when the body can actually receive and use the nutrients you eat!

PILLAR #2: ALL THE GOOD STUFF

If you are used to takeout, frozen, and restaurant meals, you are going to be so proud of yourself by the end for how well you navigate the kitchen. Every day on the ARC, you will be making flavorful alkaline teas, tonics, juices, smoothies, and soups. If you have never made soup before, you are in for an amazing experience; it's so easy to create soulful, yummy soups that you will crave. Juicing is a revelation for most newbies, too—you only need to throw in a bunch of ingredients and out comes a colorful, glowing-with-nutrients drink. Smoothies are simply a matter of flipping the blender switch, and you are rewarded with a tasty, belly-filling concoction.

Price-conscious people should know: You will spend around $175 on ingredients for the Cleanse. That's seven "meals" per day for seven days, or roughly $3.50 per meal. You can't do better at Taco Bell. You do need equipment (a juicer and a blender), but they're cost effective if you factor in the savings you'll have down the road on medications and doctors' bills, and you don't have to get anything fancy. If you're like most of my previously diet-fad-following clients, you may already have the appliances in the back of a cabinet right now, gathering dust. Well, take them out, clean them off, and make room for them by putting the coffeemaker and toaster in the cabinet for a while. As a client once told me, "If you have a juicer on the counter, you will use it. You are your accessible appliances!"

With seven "meals" or more per day, you'll never feel hungry. You need the every-two-hours eating schedule to constantly flood your body with nutrients and keep up the detoxification momentum. Don't worry about preparation, though. You will only "cook" two or three times a day. Remember, the über-pillar is "fun and easy." The teas and tonics involve little more than boiling water. Otherwise, you only have to make one batch of juice, one big smoothie, and one big soup a day. At each "preparation time," you simply make twice as much as you need— you make two servings, so you have one right away and save the other for a later meal. This halves your prep and cleaning time. And you'll never have to scrub a greasy pan. All you have to do is rinse out the juicer, blender, and pot.

People often ask, "If a juice is just a liquified salad, then why not eat the salad?" Why all the liquid and semiliquids and no "solid" food? Consuming just liquids for seven days really does give your body—especially your digestive system—a huge break and a chance to rebuild. It's *so* important that you don't fall into the trap of eating regular (albeit healthy) meals during the Cleanse. If you trigger your digestive system into having to process solid foods just once, it affects it for the whole day.

The other piece of the puzzle is that liquids bring the nutrients where they need to go faster, with a higher potential for absorption and little waste. Juices are an incredibly efficient and effective nutrient delivery system. You can pack *a lot* more nourishment into a juice than you could eat in a sitting. For example, look at the ingredients in the Triple A Juice (one of my favorites):

TRIPLE A JUICE

Makes 2 servings

Ingredients

2 handfuls of spinach	1 inch turmeric
1 handful of kale	½ red bell pepper
½ cucumber	1 small beet
1 celery stick	1 carrot
½ inch gingerroot	Filtered water to taste

Instructions

Place all the ingredients in a juicer. Process and enjoy!

You might be able to eat all that as a salad, but it would take a while. The quantity of juice this recipe yields will take you one minute to drink. You'll have this in the morning, and most people aren't able to eat or feel inclined to have that much food before rushing to work. But they'll down a juice, no problem. Juicing gives you the opportunity to transform your health rapidly, infusing your body with such an abundance of nutrients to heal effortlessly from within. You do lose the fiber, but that actually helps you. The nutrients don't have to be removed from the fiber in the digestive process. This way, they go straight into the cells and organs that need them the most.

Besides, you will be getting plenty of fiber in smoothies and soups!

I love smoothies. I don't want you to think of them as pulpy juices. They are different tools in your box. Granted, juices and smoothies on the Cleanse do have many of the same ingredients, with a few key distinctions. For one, you can't blend celery or carrots, so they will be in most of your juices. For another, you can't juice an avocado. Avo will be the foundation for most of your smoothies. Other smoothie-only ingredients include coconut oil, almonds, cashews, pumpkin and sunflower seeds, and chia seeds. In smoothies, you can enjoy a range of textures with a great variety in ingredients. Plus, fiber. Smoothies fill you up and keep you satisfied for a while. The blending also allows you to take in more nutrient-dense foods than you'd be able to chew and eat raw in one sitting, or even fit on a plate.

The last component, soup, is where the love comes in like a warm hug. If I do say so myself, my soups are beautifully filling, satisfying, warming, comforting bowls of joy. They also give you some subtle chunkiness to chew, a new texture, and the psychological magic of sitting down with a bowl and a spoon. While not all the soups on the ARC are 100 percent liquefied, those that aren't (like my hugely popular Immune-Boosting Soup and Soothing Gut-Healing Soup) are very gently chunky. They are still so gentle on your digestive system, allowing it to rest, heal, and regenerate. In fact, these are the secret weapon in the toolbox because for several hours after consuming one of these soups, you will forget you're even on a cleanse. Ingredient-wise, soups allow for even more variety, such as healthy fats, more fiber, and plant proteins like lentils and beans that you wouldn't want to put in a smoothie. More variety means abundance, high volume vitamins and minerals, and macro- and micronutrients. Some of the soups are warm, but never piping hot. Cooking foods does rob them of some of their nutrients, and consuming hot or cold food requires energy from your body in order to regulate temperature. By consuming only cool or warm foods, you're giving your body a break.

Quantity *and* Quality

Hearing that the ARC is all liquid, some clients have expressed concern that they'll feel hungry. I promise you, you'll consume *plenty* of food, and within those meals, you'll feel full, satisfied, and energized throughout the day and get more than adequate levels of protein, fat, fiber, and all your essential nutrients. If anything, you'll feel like you're eating too much and too often, rather than too little and not frequently enough.

After I explain the quantity of food on the Cleanse, some clients then worry that they'll gain weight on it. The amount of fat your body retains is a matter of balance, especially in your endocrine system. Weight gain is 80 percent caused by how effectively your hormones are interacting, definitely *not* by the volume of veggies you eat. Lean people shouldn't worry, either. Being underweight is as much a state of imbalance as being overweight is. The ARC will move you toward your perfect, ideal weight, whether that means dropping unneeded fat cells *or* adding muscle and healthy fat cells to your body.

Furthermore, you will get adequate calories per day to maintain a robust metabolic rate. Most chronic dieters know that if you are on a super-low-calorie plan, your metabolism slows to a crawl until you can eat next to nothing and still not lose fat. You don't want that to happen, and you won't come close on the ARC. The Cleanse will bring your metabolic rate to your perfect level. You provide the tools, and your body does the rest.

You will eat throughout the day, many times, to keep those metabolic fires blazing, including teas, fat-rich tonics, two or three juices, two or three smoothies, and two or three large soups, all filling and deliciously satisfying.

Rest assured, feeling hungry is *not* going to be an issue.

PILLAR #3: NONE OF THE BAD STUFF

This pillar is self-explanatory. You're going to have to completely stop your intake of any food, drink, or substance that perpetuates body imbalance. Anything that bogs down the liver, kidneys, stomach, intestines, pancreas, or adrenals cannot pass through your lips or enter your bloodstream.

That means zero acidic, inflammatory, oxidative stress-inducing foods. No meat from any creature that walks, crawls, swims, or flies. No by-products of any creature, like eggs, milk, yogurt, or cheese. No fruit except for lemons, limes, avocados, and tomatoes, which are all alkaline-forming. (I know blueberries are antioxidant powerhouses, but on the Cleanse, you are avoiding all fructose for a week. When it's over, add berries to your gluten-free oatmeal.) Also, no sugars from honey, agave, stevia, or maple syrup. *No grains.* Just none. The only acceptable oils for the week of the Cleanse are flax and coconut (with the odd drizzle of olive oil on some soups, but never heated).

Also, zero acidic, inflammatory, oxidative stress-inducing beverages like soda, seltzer, coffee, and tea (caf or decaf), hot chocolate, fruit juices, beer, wine, and cocktails. Ideally, you will *only* drink filtered water (more on that in Pillar #5), herbal teas, organic coconut water, organic coconut milk, organic almond milk, and *that is it.*

And zero acidic, inflammatory, oxidative stress-inducing substances. No smoking cigarettes or anything else. No vaping. No recreational drugs. Ideally, no OTC drugs.

A Note on Medications

Of course, I am not your doctor, physician, or consultant, and you should approach any new dietary plan with their blessing and guidance on how to continue your agreed-upon medication regimen. Taking prescribed medications should always be discussed with your health-care professional.

However, for OTC drugs, if these are optional, I do encourage you to think about their use during the Cleanse. There is no doubt that they are acidic and stressful to the body.

If you are tempted to use OTC drugs like acetaminophen/paracetamol on the Cleanse because of a temporary detox symptom like a headache, please try as hard as possible not to. This will only prolong that detox symptom, while masking it, and it will return later. When you're on the ARC, refer back to the suggestions on how to overcome detox symptoms (info on page 152) rather than masking them with OTC medications.

Pillar #4: Trust in Nature

Something that really bugs me about a lot of cleanse or detox programs is their reliance on supplements and miracle, magic-bullet products. I kind of agree with skeptics who say that people who overuse them have the most expensive urine in the world, implying that all the money you spend at the health food store is being peed away.

The fact is, you don't need pricey supplements when the goodness in whole natural foods is so ridiculously abundant. On the ARC, you just need nature.

The clue with supplements is in the name. They are there to *supplement* a healthy diet, not substitute for one. I do recommend some supplements, but they are all from nature (like green powder and psyllium husks) or ingredients you'll already consume on the Cleanse but in higher doses (like coconut oil and turmeric), and which are meant to enhance your body's ability to receive the waterfall of nourishment. In the week afterward, you can continue to add these ingredients to your diet to keep the floodgates of good health open and help you build a framework for an effortlessly abundant and energized life forever.

Of course, for some people with specific nutrient deficiencies, a short-term focus on a particular nutrient set might be needed. But don't be bamboozled by the shiny packaging or outrageous claims of certain supplements and products. Just cover the necessary basics and you'll be set.

Pillar #5: Megahydration

A nutrient that we don't often think of is water, but it is one of the most important of all. Hydration is a critical part of the protocol. One of the biggest, most common mistakes made by people on a cleanse (or at any other time!) is forgetting to drink, drink, drink. You won't be able to reach any health goal if you are dehydrated day in, day out.

Minimum daily water requirements on the Cleanse: two to four liters (roughly 100 ounces) of filtered water Every. Single. Day. I know you'll be getting lots of liquid in the water-rich, veggie-based juices, soups, and smoothies, but you have to drink the two to four liters on top of that. On the ARC, because you will be purging tons of stored acids and toxins through the liver and kidneys and out the body via urine, you need to keep the flow going (and going, and going). If you aren't sluicing away the toxins, then they'll get stuck right where they are. You're impeding your efforts if you don't drink.

What I'm saying: *You must drink!!!*

Clients have come to me in the past with two main hydration challenges:

1. Not being physically able to drink that much.

2. Not remembering to drink that much.

If you are not physically able to drink enough, start by adjusting your thinking about it. You won't sit down and drink 100 ounces of water in five minutes. If you have 16 waking hours per day, you only need to drink 6 ounces per hour. You can even work up to that level, starting with 50 ounces per day for a week (3 ounces per hour), then up to 75 ounces for a week, etc. Your body will adjust to the inflow. Think of a dried-up old sponge. When you run it under your faucet, the water bounces off and runs into the sink—at first—but even that very small amount of absorption is usable. After a short while, the sponge absorbs more. Then a little bit more. And before you know it, the sponge is able to hold and use a large volume of water before needing to be squeezed out and the process started again.

Reader, you are that sponge.

At first the water will just run straight through you, leaving you heading for the bathroom every half an hour and feeling bloated in between. But glass after glass, your body will adjust and be able to use the water, delivering it around your system and to your cells. Gradually, you will comfortably retain a lot more of the water, and the need to pee all the time will disappear. For most people, this transformation takes less than two days, and then you start to *love* drinking lots of water because of the positive effects it has on your energy, mental clarity, digestion, and skin.

As for those who forget to drink enough, I sympathize. At 9 A.M., you swear you're going to drink loads of water today, and then in a snap of your fingers, it's 9 P.M., and you've barely had any (and drinking 100 ounces a few hours before bed is not a good idea).

The human mind isn't built to remember the same information over and over throughout the day. You simply will not remember to do the same small action 10 times a day . . . unless you use my little trick.

In my previous life, I used to work for a big beverage company that made addictive products with sugar, aspartame, and additives. As if that wasn't awful enough, the company excelled in hooking people to their drinks behaviorally, too. They were experts in addiction. The best foolproof way to get someone to repeat actions over the course of the day—in their case, drink one of their drinks every few hours—was to link the new behavior to an existing habit. In this case, they linked their various beverages with meal time, break time, social time, sports, and post-exercise. People came to associate having their drinks with daily activities, and a new habit was formed.

I'm asking you to start linking water with things you do every day to form a new, healthy habit. Can you think of five or six things you do every day? Waking up and getting out of bed, brushing your teeth, preparing breakfast, arriving at work, having lunch, getting home from work, preparing dinner, brushing your teeth before bed, and so on.

If you start linking a glass of water to each of these existing activities, you'll have the habit of hydration in no time. Add a couple cups of herbal tea, like peppermint, chamomile, turmeric, ginger, or lemongrass, and you'll easily reach 100 ounces.

This is critical during the ARC. Skipping hydration during the Cleanse is counterproductive. I'd even say that it's not worth doing the Cleanse at all. Hydration moves out the toxins. It also moves along your digestive system. If you don't sluice out those systems, you just won't get the benefits.

Now, on to the important subject of the water itself.

Ideally, you'd have alkaline water, which is a huge subject and a whole book's worth of material, but I don't want to get off topic too far. If you have a source of making alkaline water, be it an ionizer, pH drops, or a filtration system, great. Continue to use it. If you don't, no worries. *But* I strongly advise you to filter your water. It's not enough to just drink 100 ounces straight from the tap. Bottled water isn't good enough either, I'm afraid. Tap water and bottled water are *full* of toxins, plus they're acidic, oxidizing, and inflammatory, and counterproductive to the aims of the Cleanse.

In 2013, the Environmental Working Group (EWG) published a report[4] on its analysis of nearly 20 million drinking water tests conducted by water suppliers nationwide between 2004 and 2009. The study revealed hundreds of pollutants in U.S. tap water. They detected 316 contaminants in water supplied to the public, including 204 chemicals, 97 agricultural pollutants, 86 contaminants

---

4   If you'd like to read more about it, go to: https://www.ewg.org/tapwater/state-of-american-drinking-water.php.

linked to pollution and treatment plants, and 42 pollutants that leached from pipes and storage tanks. It's disgusting, but not too surprising.

People were shocked by the reports in 2014 of lead contamination of the water supply in Flint, Michigan, but this is not an isolated incident. A recent study[5] in Chicago found that 70 percent of the almost 3,000 homes tested had lead in their water supply.

The shocking news stories we hear from time to time are really the tip of the iceberg. Millions of people are drinking water that does not meet standards, and hundreds of the chemicals ingested are completely unregulated. Nobody is in charge of making sure they are kept at safe levels. These unregulated chemicals—some listed below—scare me. According to the EWG, despite the potential health risks, there is no legal limit on these chemicals—no matter how high the concentrations—in drinking water. Among them, 168 have been linked to cancer, 54 to reproductive toxicity, 67 to developmental toxicity, and 35 to immune system damage.

- **Bromochloroacetic acid** is a by-product of tap water disinfection found in the water supplied to 40 million consumers. It induces gene mutations and is associated with damage to DNA.

- **Perchlorate** is a rocket fuel ingredient, toxic to the thyroid gland, and found in water provided to 26 million people.

- **Methyl tert-butyl ether** (MTBE) is a gasoline additive and groundwater pollutant scheduled to be phased out nationwide, found in 12 million people's tap water supply. It is associated with liver and kidney damage and nervous system effects.

- **Di-n-butylphthalate**, a chemical from a group of industrial plasticizers called phthalates, was found in water used by five million people. Phthalates have been linked to birth defects and reproductive toxicity.

And what of the "regulated" toxins in tap water? The most damaging toxins are not being kept below safe standards. For example, trihalomethanes have been linked to a range of health problems—including bladder cancer, colon and rectal cancer, birth defects, low birth weight, and miscarriage—and are still present in tap water in frightening levels.

So-called safe chemicals include chlorine, chloramine, and, of course, fluoride, but the reality is, they're not safe at all. Chlorine, for one, is bleach, and has been strongly linked to an increase in birth defects. According to the

---

5   To read more about *that*, go to: http://www.chicagotribune.com/news/watchdog/ct-chicago-water-lead-contamination -20180411-htmlstory.html.

U.S. Council on Environmental Quality, the cancer risk to people who drink chlorinated water is 93 percent higher than among those whose water does not contain chlorine. Chlorine from tap water has been linked to asthma, skin conditions, increased risk of miscarriage, liver problems, and more.

Chloramine, a cousin of chlorine, is the new bleach on the block that's added to the water supply. It's a less effective disinfectant than chlorine, but it lasts longer and so is now used *alongside* chlorine to help make your water "safe." Far from it. As soon as chlorine or chloramines react with any natural matter (such as decaying vegetation in the source water), disinfection by-products (DBPs) are formed. DBPs are seriously bad news: They are more than 10,000 times more toxic than chlorine, highly carcinogenic, and linked to nervous system, respiratory, and renal problems, as well as causing cardiovascular damage.

Do you want to drink that?

I haven't gotten to fluoride yet. This chemical is a common additive to tap water in the U.S., Australia, and the U.K. Most other countries do not add fluoride to their drinking water, probably for the simple reason that a substance that hardens tooth enamel might not be so great in your delicate digestive system. According to a 500-page scientific review, fluoride is also incredibly unbalancing to your endocrine system, affecting your thyroid, adrenals, bones and more.[1] Thirty-four human studies and more than 100 animal studies link fluoride to brain damage. Children living in areas with fluoridated water have been shown to have "significantly lower IQ levels."[2] It's just terrible. I'm not sure how this can happen in our modern world, where countries as developed and smart as the U.K., U.S., and Australia continue a practice that imperils the health of the entire population.

So tap is out. Unfortunately, bottled water is definitely not the place to turn. Studies have found that up to 40 percent of bottled water is actually just tap water in a bottle.[3] To make matters worse, bottled-water companies are held to standards that are laxer than tap water! The EWG found 38 contaminants in 10 brands of bottled water, including caffeine, toxic bacteria, carcinogenic DBPs, nitrates, arsenic, various industrial chemicals, and pharmaceutical agents.[4]

And then it gets worse.

Many bottles themselves are made from plastic that contains bisphenol A, more commonly known as BPA, which has been proven to leech into the water over time and in certain conditions. Those bottles sit in a warehouse for weeks and months, exposed to heat, light, and air, which happen to be the *exact* conditions under which BPA leeches into the water. In order to enjoy all these toxins and chemicals and contribute plastic to landfills and ocean pollution, you will pay a premium price—50 to 100 times what you'd pay for tap water.

Instead of buying bottles, buy a filtration system to clean your tap water. Any countertop pitcher water filter—available online for around $25—is fine to start off. They pretty much clean tap water of chlorine, chloramines, bacteria, sediment, lead, and other metals pretty well. If you want to upgrade to an installed filtration system, you have many excellent options. It is more of a financial commitment, though. I've written extensively about this and have made recommendations on my website. Go to www.rossbridgeford.com/arc for more info and guidance there.

Along with clean, clear water, you can always squeeze a lemon into it (in fact, this is a great way to start the day), and enjoy herbal teas (nothing caffeinated; steer away from green, black, and white teas) like chamomile, rooibos, lemongrass, ginger, peppermint, nettle, turmeric, or any blend you like. You will feel like you're floating down a babbling mountain-clean stream on this Cleanse, and, in a way, you will be.

The Five Pillars at a Glance

Pillar #1: Nourish, Not Punish. This is not a detox. It's not about restriction or pain. It's about giving your body what it needs to repair and reboot.

Pillar #2: All of the Good Stuff. You'll get so much healthy, delicious food, you will not believe how full you are.

Pillar #3: None of the Bad Stuff. Prepare for a sober week with no caffeine, drugs, sugar, grain, meat, and dairy.

Pillar #4: Trust in Nature. Everything you need is already in the glass or bowl, so don't worry about pills and powders.

Pillar #5: Megahydration. Rinse your body clean from the inside out. On top of the juices, smoothies, and soups, drink a minimum of 100 ounces of *filtered* water per day.

Your Alkaline Reset Cleanse Resources

Don't forget to head to www.rossbridgeford.com/arc for all your bonus resources, including my full guides for making alkaline water and the best equipment to use for filtration and making juices, smoothies, and soups.

CHAPTER 7

IT'S ALL
ABOUT RESULTS

While it is true that one person's results will not be 100 percent replicated in someone else, many common themes do come up among my ARC clients. These men and women come from all walks of life, with all different backgrounds, facing different challenges. But they are all thrilled with the results they experienced going through the ARC.

My program is highly personal, and I work one-on-one with people who sign up for the program online, with regular group chats and hangouts, and lots of questions going back and forth. It's been my greatest joy, apart from my family, to work so closely with my clients! Often, I get groups of Cleansers via Facebook to start on the same day and go through the process together, creating group support along with my individual guidance. I've gotten to know my clients very well, and they share everything they're experiencing at every step along the way. It is amazing to form such a close relationship with them and to learn from their journey. Many of my clients have been through two, three, five Cleanses with me, and it's a testimony to how powerful it is that they want to do it again and again!

If the results weren't what they hoped for, they would dump me and my program in a heartbeat. But the results *are* fantastic, which is why they keep coming back for more. They feel deeply connected with their bodies, energized, and full of vitality, strength, and confidence. Feeling that incredible is, well, a bit addictive! When you feel that good, you don't ever want to feel tired and wiped out again.

Benefits of the ARC

As you do the Cleanse and balance the Five Master Systems, you will notice that your body will start to show improvement in every single way, in every single cell.

- Healing of inflammation
- No more pain
- No more swelling
- No more fatigue
- Reduction of excess fat
- Lifting of mood
- Sustaining of energy all day
- Easing of autoimmune conditions (lupus, rheumatoid arthritis, polymyalgia)
- No more skin conditions (psoriasis, eczema, rosacea)
- Improvement of digestive conditions (acid reflux, Crohn's, IBS)
- Better sleep
- Cleared thinking
- Growth in bone strength
- Improvement of liver and kidney function
- Strengthening of immunity

The improvements from the ARC are the result of correcting global imbalances. Other methods attempt to address a specific symptom.

Take fatigue, for example. Why are you so tired all the time?

Well, it could be adrenal fatigue, a common cause of low energy in our chronically stressed-out world.

It could be flattened microvilli in the small intestine or candida overgrowth hogging nutrients and clogging your digestive tract, preventing absorption that every cell in your body requires, causing brain fog, headaches, and tiredness.

Maybe you have poor insulin response due to years of sugar and wheat consumption, and your pancreas is overwhelmed, causing wild blood sugar dips and spikes.

Or your liver and kidneys aren't functioning properly due to the stresses of the standard modern diet, chronic dehydration, and a stagnant lymphatic system.

Or an overactive autoimmune response has impaired your thyroid function.

You get my point. If you attempted to fix one issue for a certain benefit, it might work in the short term. But if you want long-term solutions to widespread, multipronged problems, you need a holistic approach. The beauty of the ARC is that it fixes everything simultaneously—your adrenals and thyroid, blood sugar spikes, cortisol, leptin, and ghrelin. It heals and seals the gut, cutting off the source of autoimmune diseases at the root. And, of course, it gives your body an avalanche of easily digested nourishment so that all your hungry cells—from your brain to your skeleton to every muscle and fiber—feels energized and alive.

By rebalancing, cleansing, and nourishing the FMS, you will get results quickly, powerfully, and for the long term.

Denise's Story

When I think back to my reason for starting the Cleanse, it goes back to when I got a virus that wouldn't go away. I felt really low energy for a month, and then a month later, I noticed a swelling in my fingers that got worse and worse. It was very painful and looked awful.

And then it spread to my back and neck. All of a sudden I couldn't move freely and most of my day was spent in pain. After seeing the doctor, I was diagnosed with psoriatic arthritis. They told me the only answer was a lifetime of medication and to expect it to get worse as time went on. I was so scared and felt so hopeless, but worse, the medication didn't work.

I'd followed Ross's alkaline eating before and it had worked for me then to increase my energy. I knew I needed something more powerful this time. I had to do it in a big way, so I joined his Alkaline Reset Cleanse program.

After just the first "reset," the difference was amazing. My energy was unrecognizable. I actually felt *well* again, full of life. Waking up early and not feeling tired from the moment I got up was just fantastic. I'd get home from work still energized despite being on my feet all day.

The inflammation and pain subsided straightaway, and everything started to come together. The fact that my energy came back, that my neck, back, and joints were pain-free again, was enough incentive. This was going to be for life.

Within just a few months, I completely stopped taking medication. I went to see the consultant who did all the X-rays and blood exams, and everything came back clear. I am completely free of arthritis!

Over the course of the week before, the week during, and the week after the Cleanse, I lost more than 15 pounds. Now I'm back to how much I weighed before I had children in my early 20s!

My psoriasis has also gone, which has been a real life-changer, too. It used to be quite debilitating and depressing when it flared up, but no more. That's just another amazing thing the ARC has given me. But really, it's given me back my life. Feeling fit, feeling healthy, having a level of energy I never thought I'd see again. There is just no substitute for how I feel now.

Robert's Story

About 27 years ago, I was diagnosed with polycystic kidneys, and the prognosis was that my kidney function would reduce more and more over my life until I needed a transplant. It left me with increasing symptoms of pain, fatigue, frequent infections, and lots of inflammation.

Now I've got three beautiful children, a 14-year-old daughter and twin 12-year-old girls. The kids are a handful, just *full on!* The twins have autism, so life is often very, very busy.

I knew I had a serious health problem when the twins were about six. One morning, after spending 45 minutes just trying to get the kids to school and feeling exhausted, by the time we finally got there, we were an hour late. As I walked them in, I knew I needed help. I remember thinking, *I can't go on like this.*

I started looking for answers, but nothing has really worked—until I found Ross.

When I first started, all I did was have smoothies for breakfast. I thought, *This can't be enough*, but it was! Little changes like that, one change at a time—a juice here, a smoothie there—it wasn't hard at all. It gave me hope and an entirely different feeling. So I added more.

The energy I have now, I can't describe it, it's just an amazing feeling. Having two or three of the juices or smoothies a day meant my energy just didn't end! For the first time in my life, I felt awake and good when I woke up, and just as good at the end of the day when I went to bed!

I'd been told by my doctor I would *always* have pain and that my joints were "worn out." I never wanted to believe this, and I was right not to. Now I have no more pain. My joints aren't aching anymore, and my skin has cleared! I always had pretty bad rosacea. My face was red and blotchy and I had pimples that wouldn't go away, but now it's all gone.

Since my energy came back, I started running, and it felt great. I met someone who said I should try a half marathon, so I signed up for that and loved it. And then someone told me, "If you can do a half, you can do a whole."

I'd always wanted to do that, and mentioned it at my annual appointment with my kidney specialist. He said, "Absolutely don't do that!" I asked why, and he told me, "Healthy people die running marathons and you've got polycystic kidneys!"

It only made me more determined, and soon after, I ran my first marathon.

I can't tell you the difference the ARC has made to my life. Before, I couldn't walk 40 yards up my driveway to fetch the mail, and now I'm running marathons. Instead of looking forward to a life of less and less energy, all I can see now is energy whenever I want for as long as I want. I'm just getting stronger and stronger every day. I have to say, I'm pretty excited about life again.

Val's Story

I'm a 53-year-old mother of two in New York City. I did the ARC to lose weight since I've tried every other diet and failed every time. I broke out the juicer (from the time I juiced for one day and got bored), my Magic Bullet blender (from the time I smoothied for one day and hated it), and my soup pot (from the soup diet that left my kitchen a disaster site and made my family rebel against me). I timed the Cleanse to a week when my kids and husband were out of town on vacation. I'd stayed home to take care of the cats and meet a deadline, so I was alone with my juicer and blender for the entire seven days.

I followed the recipes to the letter at first, and then made some minor adjustments to the protocol along the way. For one thing, I couldn't drink two smoothies a day. It was just too much food. So I would make the smoothie in the afternoon, have one portion then, and the second portion for breakfast the next day, a slight deviation from Ross's plan. I am not a watercress fan, so I substituted that ingredient with spinach. Little tweaks like that. I kept to the Five Pillars, though, and had only liquids, and didn't touch coffee or alcohol at all.

I had some ups and downs during the Cleanse, like caffeine-withdrawal headaches, some queasiness, some aches and pains. I didn't miss coffee as much as I thought I would. By Day Five, I felt pretty good! My best day was Day Seven. I finished the Cleanse strong, on a high note. I felt energetic, but I hadn't lost much weight.

And then, as the days went on, funny things started happening. A couple of days post-Cleanse, I had to tighten my belt a notch, and another a few days later. My psoriasis was clearing on its own without creams. The thumbnail that always split at a certain length? It doesn't do that anymore. There's less hair in the shower drain after a shampoo. My gums stopped bleeding when I brushed them. When I cut my finger while chopping veggies, it didn't bleed nearly as much as other, similar cuts, and it never swelled up. And this was truly weird: It healed *so fast*. Like, vampire fast. My sleep was the most pleasant surprise. I have struggled with insomnia for decades. Nearly every night, I would lie awake for two or three hours, anxiety-ridden about how tired I was going to be the next day. I have been amazed how quickly I nod off now, and how deeply I'm sleeping. I'm well rested every morning, and the anxiety related to my insomnia is gone. I'm not afraid to get in bed anymore.

By the end of the post-Cleanse week, I'd lost six pounds (all in the belly, it seems), and felt like I'd not only reset my master systems, but my entire way of eating and outlook on life.

I am so passionate about this Cleanse, so grateful I attained the knowledge, skills, and instincts to create it, and so humbled and happy to get to teach it and guide people on this path. This is my calling. It changes lives, and I share gratitude daily for the opportunity I have been given to help improve the lives of others through good health.

Life is nothing without our health.

Health is freedom, the greatest freedom.

Now you will begin your own success story, and make large strides, notice big and small changes in your health, and take that harmony and energy into your work and relationships.

Next up, a very specific guide to the foods you will be eating on the Cleanse and how their nutrients will flood your cells with goodness.

CHAPTER 8

EVERYTHING YOU'LL EAT ON THE ARC

Every meal of every day on the ARC, you will get so many vitamins, minerals, and phytonutrients, your body will absolutely *love* you and the beneficial effect will be almost instantly obvious. All the foods are Triple A approved, meaning they are all alkaline, anti-inflammatory, and antioxidant. They are the most nutrient-dense foods on earth.

In 2014, researchers at William Paterson University compiled a list[1] of the world's most healthful foods. They looked at each food's nutrient density and bioavailability, awarding "powerhouse" status for fruits and veggies that provided, on average, 10 percent or more of the RDA of 17 nutrients (including fiber, potassium, protein, calcium, folate, and vitamins A, B_{12}, and D) that have been proven to prevent and reverse chronic disease. Of the top 41, 38 are alkaline-forming foods, the top 16 of which are leafy greens.

Powerhouse Veggies and Fruits

- Watercress
- Chinese cabbage
- Chard
- Beet greens
- Spinach
- Chicory

- Leaf lettuce
- Parsley
- Romaine lettuce
- Collard greens
- Turnip greens
- Mustard greens

- Endive
- Chive
- Kale
- Dandelion greens
- Red pepper
- Arugula
- Broccoli
- Pumpkin
- Brussels sprouts
- Scallion
- Kohlrabi
- Cauliflower
- Cabbage
- Carrot
- Tomato
- Lemon
- Iceberg lettuce
- Strawberry
- Radish
- Winter squash
- Orange
- Lime
- Pink grapefruit
- Rutabaga
- Turnip
- Blackberry
- Leek
- Sweet potato
- White grapefruit

To become a health powerhouse, you need to eat an abundance of power-house foods—in particular, the most potent leafy greens. However, if you ate only the above foods, you wouldn't get adequate fat and protein in your diet. To address those nutritional needs, the ARC has seeds, nuts, nut milks, oils, and legumes to round things out. I'll bet you've at least tried most of these foods before—nothing scary or weird here! And you can consume the foods in the ARC with wild abandon.

The Alkaline Reset Cleanse foods include:

Almonds

Almond milk

Arugula

Avocado

Basil

Beets (with beet greens)

Bell peppers (red and green)

Broccoli

Butternut squash

Cabbage (all varieties)

Cannellini beans

Carrots

Cashews

Celery

Chard

Chia seeds

Cilantro

Coconut milk and cream

Coconut oil

Coconut water

Collard greens

Cucumber

Dill

Garlic

Ginger

Kale

Lentils

Lettuce (all varieties)

Leek

Lemons

Limes

Olive oil

Onion (yellow and red)

Parsley

Pumpkin

Scallions

Spices and seasonings (cayenne, black pepper, Himalayan salt, sea salt, nutmeg, mustard seeds, vanilla pods)

Spinach

Sunflower seeds

Sweet potato

Tea (herbal)

Tomato

Turmeric

Vegetable stock

Water (filtered)

Watercress

Foods to *avoid* on the Alkaline Reset Cleanse
Everything else

Seriously, Back-Away-Slowly Foods

Animal protein

Bread (pastry, cakes, cookies)

Caffeinated drinks (coffee, tea, soda)

Carbonated drinks (anything with bubbles, including seltzer)

Dairy (milk, cheese, yogurt, cream)

Chocolate

Condiments

Honey

Fast foods

Fruit

Gluten-containing grains (wheat, rye, spelt, freekeh)

Mushrooms

Pasta

Processed foods

Refined foods

Sugar

Sugar substitutes

Sweets

Vegetable oil

Vinegar

Yeast-containing products

Your Alkaline Reset Cleanse Resources

For a full list of 400-plus ranked acid/alkaline foods and guide to the Healthiest Sugar Alternatives, go to www.rossbridgeford.com/arc.

The problem with fruit, as delicious and nutritious as it is, is that it contains fructose, a sugar.

Fructose can be a huge problem.

Humans were not designed to eat vast volumes of fructose, not only from fruit but from other sources as well. Many sugars—table, brown, raw, cane—are 50 percent glucose, 50 percent fructose. Other sugars—maple syrup, honey, agave, molasses—also contain some fructose. Fructose is also an additive in nearly every processed food. The worst offender is high-fructose corn syrup, which accounts for at least half the fructose consumed on average, particularly in the U.S.

Fructose is a stealth bomb. Although glucose is acidic, inflammatory, oxidizing, and what I consider to be bad news all around, every cell of the body makes use of it in moderate amounts. The trouble with fructose is that it can *only* be metabolized by the liver. Many new clients tell me that they eat well because of all the apples and oranges they eat. Unfortunately, all that fructose has stressed out their liver and pancreas (the insulin-producing gland). A stressed-out liver and pancreas translate into a host of issues that many of my fruit-loving clients have to contend with, such as:

- **Insta-inflammation.** When sugar melts with protein, it undergoes the Maillard reaction. Imagine melting butter in a pan and then adding sugar. What do you get? A browned, sticky, gooey syrup. The same reaction takes place *inside* the body, and the resulting caramelized gunk is the perfect breeding ground for what's known as superoxide free radicals to flourish. Not only that, but when the liver itself is inflamed, it inhibits amino acid (a protein building block) quality, and protein synthesis (the creation of protein required to perform nearly every bodily function).

- **Increased fat-cell production.** When fructose enters the liver, a process called lipogenesis begins. Lipogenesis is exactly what it sounds like: the creation of new fat cells. According to a recent study by researchers at the University of California, Davis, two groups of overweight subjects were given beverages containing glucose, but only one group's drink also contained fructose. At the end of the study period, both groups gained weight, but the fructose group gained significantly more visceral fat volume.[2]

- **Increased risk of type 2 diabetes.** A recent review study published in the *Journal of Nutrition & Food Sciences* looked at more than 150 published studies and pinpointed fructose (both natural and processed high-fructose corn syrup) as the leading risk factor in developing type 2 diabetes.[3] Furthermore, research out of the Mayo Clinic implicated fructose as the "greatest problem for diabetes,

diabetes related abnormalities, and cardiovascular risk."[4] Type 2 diabetes—and its related complications—is a leading cause of mortality in the Western world, just behind cancer, stroke, and cardiovascular disease. Cutting fructose directly cuts the risk, dramatically.

- **Destabilized hunger hormones.** The two hormones that are primarily responsible for our hunger and satiety are leptin and ghrelin. When your liver is bombarded with fructose, these two hunger hormones are thrown out of balance. As a result, you feel always hungry and never full.

In some ways, fruit is just as bad, if not worse in some circumstances, than a candy bar. For one, because it's natural and healthy, people assume they can eat as much fruit as they want without harming themselves. *Not true.* You'd never sit down and eat 10 candy bars, but you might not hesitate to eat 10 servings of grapes or 10 small clementines. I'm not saying you can never have fruit again, or that it is solely or directly responsible for all the problems I've just mentioned. But the truth about fructose is that it's not "healthy." You just can't eat fruit—in any form, be it whole, juiced, or blended—with abandon, especially if you are prediabetic or diabetic.

While you are doing the seven days of the ARC, you won't have any fruit. None in the juices or smoothies, at all. After the Cleanse, I recommend one to two pieces a day, and quitting fruit juice for good, whether it's made fresh or store-bought. Dumping that much fructose into the body is catastrophic to the liver. Apologies to the state of Florida, but it's a crime that orange juice is touted as good for you; the truth is more like the opposite. When the fiber is removed from the fruit, the fructose is more rapidly metabolized, throwing your liver immediately into distress mode. Dried fruits are just as damaging. They're like regular fruit, concentrated. I don't allow fruits in smoothies because, despite the fiber, you drink a smoothie faster than you'd eat the fruit, which also taxes the liver.

The exceptions to the no-fruit rule are lemons, limes, tomatoes, and avocados. They contain practically zero fructose and are rich in alkaline minerals, antioxidants, and anti-inflammatory compounds.

Why Are Lemons Alkaline?

When I explain the ARC to people, I often get questions like, "Lemons are acidic, so why are they on the Cleanse?" and "The stomach is acidic, so what's the point of eating alkaline foods?"

These are very good questions. It's true that lemons are acidic. If you used a pH test strip on lemon juice, it would come back bright red (as opposed to alkaline purple). And yes, it's also true that everything we eat goes straight to the stomach, a big pool of acid that turns food into a digestible mash called chyme.

But the human body and the way it processes food is more complicated than that.

As your food enters the digestive process, it immediately prepares for digestion in the mouth with saliva, mucus, and enzymes. As the food hits the esophagus, it triggers the release of gastrin, a peptide hormone, which kick-starts the release of hydrochloric acid (HCl) in the stomach. You might have an image of your stomach as a big pouch of bubbling acid, just waiting for food to drop in and fizz and sizzle down to nothing. But this is not how it works. The stomach is usually in waiting mode, "holding" a pH of 5 to 6 (mildly acidic). When gastrin sets off the chain reaction release of HCl, the stomach's pH drops down to 4. At that level, food can be broken down and bacteria destroyed.

The amount of HCl, and just how low your stomach pH will go, depends on what you eat. An acidic diet of sugar, grains, processed foods, excessive caffeine, animal protein, dairy, processed fats, and junk food produces way too much acid, more than the body can neutralize, forcing it into survival mode, which increases inflammation and oxidative stress, all the major baddies.

Counterintuitively, an acidic diet can also make your stomach *under*produce HCl, which throws a wrench into the entire digestive process in a different way. Bear with me. The stomach creates HCl on demand. The more alkaline the food, the more stomach acid produced. To keep its digestion mode pH at 4, it has to counter the alkalizing effects of your greens with *more acid.*

Even though it sounds like a bad thing, it's not. Here's why: Whenever the stomach produces HCl, it also produces a corresponding amount of highly alkaline sodium bicarbonate (NaHCO3), essentially, baking soda. HCl and NaHCO3 both go up and down together. The more acid your stomach produces, the more alkalinity it makes, too. You need both for proper digestion. While the HCl turns your food into chyme, the NaHCO3 is passed into the bloodstream to help prepare the liver, pancreas, duodenum, and small intestine for the *next* phases of digestion. If they aren't prepared, they don't do the job of absorbing nutrients well enough.

In other words, alkaline foods ensure the stomach produces the necessary amount of acid *and* alkalinity to break down food and (later) absorb nutrients.

Acidic foods don't require the stomach to produce more HCl, and therefore, it doesn't produce enough NaHCO3 to ensure proper digestion.

Digestion is such a delicate balance. Eating acidic foods almost guarantees problems in one way or another. It can cause so much acid that the body struggles to buffer it. It can also cause too low stomach acid. Chronically low stomach acid means your food isn't broken down, which leads to undigested matter clogging the intestines and reducing absorption. You still get all the calories, though, and will get heavier and heavier, while starving cells of vital nutrients.

When you eat a diet rich in alkaline-forming foods, your stomach reacts to the increase in alkalinity with more HCl, and NaHCO3 to balance the acidity, and the upcoming harmonious, happy absorption of nutrients.

Which all brings me back to the lemon. When metabolized, its citric acid produces by-products that are highly alkalizing and that help the kidneys rid the body of excess acid via urine. So have warm lemon water every morning to start the day alkaline!

There are some levels of fructose in sweeter vegetables like carrots, beets, and sweet potatoes, and that's why even these are kept to a minimum on the ARC. You'll see small amounts of them popping up here and there, but rarely as a main ingredient in a recipe. Plus, their fructose levels are much lower than those found in the fruits.

Fructose Content of Fruits vs. Vegetables (per 100 grams)	
Fruits	**Vegetables**
Apples: 5.9 g	Beets: 0.1 g
Bananas: 4.9 g	Carrots: 0.6 g
Grapes: 8.1 g	Sweet Potatoes: 0.7 g
Pears: 6.2 g	Bell Peppers: 2.1 g
Blueberries: 5.4 g	
Strawberries: 3.3 g	

THE NUTRIENT PROFILE OF THE ALKALINE RESET

New clients are often concerned that they will miss out on certain nutrients on the Cleanse, and I totally understand why. Other cleanses or detox programs make a misguided attempt to starve out toxins. Even though on the ARC you'll be consuming far, far more nutrients than you normally would, people still worry. They hear "juices, smoothies, and soups," and think they'll be deprived of necessary proteins and fats, as if meat and dairy are the only sources of protein in the world! You will get tons of protein on the ARC from seeds, nuts, legumes, broccoli, spinach, kale, sweet potatoes, avocado, beets, carrots, and squash. You'll have multiple servings per day of at least a dozen plant proteins, more than you'll need to meet the nutritional requirement.

I'll say this about meat: It's got protein, but that's about it. Beef has some iron and vitamins B_{12} and B_6. Chicken has some B_3 and B_6, plus minerals selenium and phosphorus. Some fish is high in vitamin D and omega-3 fatty acids, which is good. But many also contain mercury, which is very bad. Compared to veggies, nuts, seeds, oils, and legumes, meat just isn't up to the task. After the Cleanse, many clients reintroduce meat into their diet. Many find that their appetite for meat has diminished and find themselves veering toward plants more and more, until the animal portion on the plate is negligible.

As for dairy, the whole thing about drinking milk to grow strong bones is a total myth. Multiple studies have proven that a habit of drinking cow's milk can actually weaken, not strengthen, bones in humans, because—irony of ironies—it leeches calcium *out* of bones. The reason for this? First of all, the calcium in dairy is poorly absorbed in our digestive system. Studies show that less than 30 percent of the calcium in milk is actually absorbed (compared to up to 65 percent of the calcium in veggies).[5] But mainly, milk, like all animal products, is acid forming.

One of the body's alkalizing forces is calcium. Where does the body go to find calcium to buffer dairy-induced acid? *Your own bones.* When consumed by humans of all ages, cow's milk, made for baby cows, is a net-calcium *loss.* A 12-year study[6] of nearly 78,000 middle-aged women found that a lifetime of consuming dairy doesn't protect women from developing osteoporosis or hip fractures. In fact, it *increases* the risk of brittle bones, fractures, and mortality in both women and men! In adolescents and children, the risk is even more alarming. A 2012 study showed that adolescent girls who consumed the most dairy were at the greatest risk of fractures in later life.[7]

Plus, dairy contains the sugars lactose and D-galactose, which cause sugar-related problems, like insulin resistance, digestive issues, oxidative stress, and weight gain. Researchers have known this since the 1990s, but the incorrect message still gets out there. It's not hard to imagine why. Big Food puts profits before health.

What foods are high in calcium that *is* absorbed and *doesn't* rob the bones? They're on the ARC: chia, spinach, kale, almonds, beans, and broccoli.

Nutrition is much bigger than macronutrients protein, fat, carbohydrates, and fiber. On the ARC, your intake of both macro- and micronutrients—such as calcium; magnesium; potassium; vitamins A, B, C, D, E, and K; and phytonutrients like carotenoids and flavonoids—will be huge. The menu is well rounded with antioxidant-rich, anti-inflammatory, alkaline, chlorophyll-rich, sulforaphane-rich, and vitamin- and mineral-rich foods, providing an abundance of nutrients you would not normally have had consistently on, say, a high-protein diet or the standard modern diet.

Snapshot of Nutrient Intake from Day Five of the Alkaline Reset Cleanse	
Nutrient	**Recommended Dietary Intake %**
Protein	228%
Vitamin A	2873%
Vitamin C	1398%
Vitamin E	138%
Vitamin K	8022%
Niacin	117%
Thiamin	243%
Riboflavin	187%
Vitamin B$_6$	294%
Folate	757%
Pantothenic Acid	128%
Calcium	150%
Iron	302%
Magnesium	325%
Phosphorus	220%
Potassium	314%
Zinc	98%
Copper	239%
Manganese	737%

As you can see, you're getting everything you need in abundance. And don't worry about "overconsuming" any nutrient. Not only is this level of nutrient intake very gentle on the body when the vitamins and minerals are from natural sources, but virtually all of these nutrients are either used or eliminated by the body—there are no toxic levels of naturally derived vitamin K, for example. It's a flood of good stuff that is all your body needs to rebalance, reboot, and reset.

CHAPTER 9

ARC SUPPLEMENTS AND SUPPLIES

Food is medicine and medicine is food. I believe that with all my heart. But you can give natural medicine a leg up with a few extra items—specifically, supplements (just a few!) and kitchen equipment. Everything I recommend in this chapter will help you get the most out of the Cleanse, and you will be happy to have it going forward once the Cleanse is over. I would never have you go out and buy something that I didn't know with absolute certainty would be of great value to you and your family long term.

SUPPLEMENTS

Many people are overwhelmed by the very idea of supplements. There are so many out there, and all of them make amazing promises. I have only one rule about them: Supplements are there to *supplement*, not replace.

I cannot reiterate this enough. This rule is especially true on the ARC, when you will be getting such an abundance of nutrients from real, whole foods. But, just to be sure you have a safety net and that nothing is missed, I do recommend a few extra helpers. For those who already have a supplement regimen that you're happy with, just stick with it. And please do consider adding my suggestions, too.

Healthy Fats

Fats are absolutely critical to human health. They've been wrongly vilified throughout our recent history and blamed for all manner of sickness and diseases *that they actually prevent*!

Healthy fats—namely, omega 3 and saturated fat (fats that are solid at room temperature)—are necessary for your brain and immune system to function, for your liver to metabolize stored fat cells, and to regulate your endocrine system. Do not worry about coconut oils, avocados, seeds, and nuts harming your heart or raising bad cholesterol! You have nothing to fear from healthy fats, at all.

So now that we've removed the fear of fat, I hope you will increase your intake with **two to three tablespoons of a high-quality omega-3 supplement per day.**

With omega oils, you get what you pay for. The brands I trust are Udo's Choice and Nordic Naturals. Generally speaking, oils should be kept in the fridge, so *do not* buy in bulk! If you see a bottle of 300 capsules for $10, assume that it's not worth even that. Expect to pay around $20 to $40 for a month's supply.

Omega-3 supplements are either fish-based (from krill or cod, usually) or plant-based (from flax and chia). Each source has a different blend of omega-3 fatty acids. For example, linolenic acid (ALA) is found in plant oils, while eicosapentaenoic acid (EPA) and docosahexaenoic acid (DHA) are found in marine oils. So I recommend a mix of fish and flax to make sure you get both.[6]

The other healthy fat I'd like you to increase is **organic coconut oil, one tablespoon per day.** Coconut oil is by far the most cost-effective way to get essential saturated fats into your diet. It contains lauric acid, myristic acid, caprylic acid, capric acid, caproic acid, palmitic acid, oleic acid, and small amounts of palmitoleic acid, linoleic acid, linolenic acid, and stearic acid. All of these saturated fats are critical for heart health, brain functioning, increasing beneficial HDL cholesterol, reducing and removing the harmful LDL cholesterol, strengthening bones and the immune system, improving liver health, lung health, reducing inflammation, balancing the endocrine system, speeding metabolism, and nourishing the skin. The lauric acid in coconut oils, specifically, has been proven to lower bad cholesterol and support cognitive function. It's also antimicrobial, so you can use it to heal, clean, and protect your skin. The caprylic acid is a powerful antibacterial and will be fantastic at destroying candida in your gut.

---

6   The bioavailability and completeness of these different fatty acids has long been debated. If you want to explore this more, I recommend *Fats That Heal, Fats That Kill* by Dr. Udo Erasmus, *Fat for Fuel* by Dr. Joseph Mercola, or *Eat Fat, Get Thin* by Dr. Mark Hyman.

Coconut oil is really an all-purpose wonder. You could survive on a desert island if you ate nothing but. If it were cost effective, I'd tell people to bathe in it!

Another good fat to consider is MCT oil, either in place of or along with coconut oil. MCT (medium chain triglycerides) oils are very similar to coconut oil, but with the lauric acid removed, and a higher concentration of caproic acid, caprylic acid, and capric acid. People in sports and bodybuilding prefer MCT oils because they are believed to help increase muscle mass. It's also more refined, and therefore more expensive. The choice is totally up to you. Either coconut or MCT or a combination; just make sure you get one tablespoon per day, in addition to the oil you'll use when making the ARC recipes.

Green Powder

I like to add green powder to my Cleanse regimen for a few reasons. First, it's just bursting with nutrients that top up the nutrients you're getting from the ARC. Second, it flavors the water you'll be drinking throughout the day and adds a little extra sustenance to the hydration part of the ARC. A scoop per day is all you need.

When shopping for a green powder, you should look for one that is organic, non-GMO, and contains a variety of ingredients including wheatgrass, barley grass, kamut grass, kelp and other sea vegetables, and dehydrated vegetables. Avoid any green powder with acid-forming fruit, mushrooms, or algae. *Definitely* avoid any that are not naturally flavored. If you absolutely must, sweeteners luo han guo (a Chinese fruit that is very concentrated and so only a little is needed) or stevia are okay. They are not ideal, but if you use any sweeteners, they are the least harmful.

Psyllium Husk

If you suffer from digestion issues (constipation or diarrhea), I recommend psyllium husk in capsules or powder. It's really inexpensive, but a highly effective supplement for keeping things moving in a comfortable way. You need both soluble (absorbs water) and insoluble (does not absorb water) fiber in your digestion system to sweep up toxins and bad cholesterol on their way out of the body and to regulate hunger and hormones. Psyllium husk has both types, making it the perfect combo and all the additional fiber you'll need on the Cleanse.

Turmeric

Adding a good-quality turmeric supplement to your diet is a smart move. It's the most potent anti-inflammatory substance out there, especially in root form (you might also see it advertised as curcumin). Since inflammation is at the root cause of so many issues within the body, it certainly doesn't hurt to top up with *extra* turmeric powder beyond what you'll be using every day in morning teas, juices, and smoothies. The vast majority of my clients started the Cleanse with a huge degree of inflammation built up in their body, and they needed a lot of turmeric to take care of it. You won't need to keep up such a huge intake of it after the Cleanse. But during? It can yield huge results.

How to Get More Turmeric in Your Diet Every Day

Before and during the Cleanse, you will see turmeric in the majority of recipes. But don't stop there! You can add this superfood into your meals in several ways:

- **Tea** Boil filtered water (or nut milk) in a pan and add a tablespoon or two of grated turmeric root and gingerroot to the pan, simmer for 5 to 10 minutes, and serve!

- **Soups** Add powdered or grated root, in blended or nonblended soups, into your pot for extra anti-inflammatory flavor.

- **Smoothies** Blend an inch or two of turmeric root into any smoothie. Using it will keep you from throwing fruit in there, because turmeric and fruit don't generally go well together.

- **Juices** Add a pinch of turmeric in the juicer in addition to all the other ingredients.

- **Salads** Grate turmeric root into the salad just before dressing. Be warned, this will turn your fingers yellow. Use kitchen gloves to avoid this!

Alkaline Mineral Supplements

There are several good supplements on the market (in pill or drop form) that contain the powerfully **alkaline minerals** sodium, potassium, magnesium, and calcium in bicarbonate form. These minerals help buffer acids in your system that need to be removed during the Cleanse.

Alkaline protein is appropriate for anyone who exercises with intensity or resistance and is already taking a protein powder. I don't recommend that you stop using a protein supplement during the Cleanse, but it would be a good idea to switch to an alkaline source as opposed to the whey protein supplements that many people use, which is concentrated dairy and filled with highly acidic, toxic, chemical flavors and colorings. Back when I first started my alkaline journey, you couldn't find an alkaline protein powder anywhere. The closest option was soy protein isolate, which isn't dairy, but might be more acid-forming than whey! But times have changed, and now you can get amazing alkaline protein powders that are just as protein-rich as whey, weighing in at 22 to 24 grams of protein per scoop. Sprouted brown rice powders are preferable, but pea protein, quinoa, and sacha inchi are all acceptable, too. They have a great amino acid profile and are gentle on digestion, along with being mildly alkaline for a win, win, win situation!

Probiotics

Probiotics are somewhat controversial. Some cleanse experts recommend them right away, while others say not to take them. My recommendation is *not* to take them during the Cleanse. But after the Cleanse is finished, you might want to try them.

Research shows that bacteria (good or bad) feeds off bacteria (good or bad). Therefore, if you have too much bad bacteria in the gut right now, putting more bacteria in there, even if it's the good kind, will only serve to feed the bad stuff. It's like throwing gasoline on a fire, which is not the way to achieve your health goals. Make sense? Once you've reset and rejuvenated your gut environment on the Cleanse, *then* go ahead and repopulate your gut with good bacteria.

My protocol for probiotics is called Weed-Seed-Feed. Within this protocol, there's plenty of wiggle room for you to tailor it to your own needs and beliefs, so don't worry about being perfect (*never* worry about being perfect!). Here's how I do it:

Step one: *Weed*. Cut off bad bacteria's food supply by eliminating sugar and gluten from your diet for a sustained period of time. You will do this on the Cleanse.

Step two: *Seed*. After the Cleanse, while consuming your greens, healthy oils, and fresh foods, seed a whole new colony of amazing good bacteria in your gut with fermented foods like sauerkraut, kimchi, and kombucha (one to two servings a day), as well as a probiotics supplement, for two to three weeks.

Step three: *Feed* your established and thriving good bacteria colony with lots of veggies, fresh foods, and filtered water, and by continuing to avoid sugar and gluten. Stop your daily intake of fermented foods; they're acid-forming. Also, you can stop using the probiotic supplement.

Supplement List

Think quality! Do not buy in bulk. You are shooting for optimal health, not discounted.

Omega 3. Two to three tablespoons per day of a combination of marine and flax oil.

Organic coconut oil. One tablespoon per day in addition to what you'll use in ARC recipes.

MCT oils. Either in place of or in combination with coconut oil; one tablespoon per day.

Green powder. One scoop per day to add flavor to your filtered water.

Psyllium husk. One heaping teaspoon per day of powder.

Turmeric powder. One teaspoon per day of organic powdered turmeric or a supplement taken as per manufacturer instructions.

Alkaline minerals. In drops or pills, take the daily recommended dose.

Alkaline protein powder (optional). One scoop (30 grams) per day.

Probiotics. After the Cleanse is completed, take daily for two to three weeks or two servings of fermented foods per day.

Your Alkaline Reset Cleanse Resources: Supplement Buyers Guide

For a full guide to these supplements, including recommended brands and sources, go to your ARC Resources at www.rossbridgeford.com/arc.

SUPPLIES

You don't need a lot of equipment to do the Cleanse, but you will require, without question, these two items:

1. A juicer
2. A blender

To make juices, you must have a juicer. To make smoothies, you need a blender. (As for blended soups, you can use a traditional blender, but it's even easier to use an immersion blender.) Unfortunately, you can't make juice with a blender, and you can't make smoothies with a juicer, despite what some blenders' marketing teams will tell you. If the fiber is still in it, it's not a juice. Period.

If you already have these items, fantastic. You're good to go. If you don't, it is time to invest in what might be the most important and effective purchases you could possibly make for yourself. Thankfully, the price of juicers has come down a lot in recent years. You can get a decent juicer for less than $50. A good blender for smoothies runs about the same. An immersion blender (a handheld gizmo you put into liquids) for soups costs less than $30. So, for a grand total of $130, you will be fully equipped for a happy, healthy life.

Juicers

As inexpensive as a juicer can be, you want to get value for your investment. In my experience, the midrange juicers are not substantially better than the cheaper ones, so while you're waiting for an expensive brand to go on sale or saving up for one, just go budget. Perfectly adequate $50 to $100 juicers can be found at a variety of retailers. It won't last for years and years, but it will give you a good 12 to 18 months of daily use before it conks out. I recommend two brands—Hurom and Kuvings—that are more expensive—but again, if you can't afford one of these, do not worry! Just go cheap.

There are two types of juicers:

Centrifugal juicers are generally less expensive and a bit less efficient. How it works: You put the vegetable into a chute, which connects to a barbed basket that spins rapidly, grating the veggie to extract the juice. It works, but it does destroy some of the nutrients in the process, and the juice doesn't stay fresh for quite as long. Also, cleaning it is a bit of a pain.

Masticating juicers use a slow gear to crush, squash, and squish the juice out of the vegetable. It's more gentle, but a little slower. The benefits are that it extracts a *lot* more juice from the vegetable, the nutrients are kept intact, and the juice will last a lot longer. It's also way easier to clean.

The juicer sitting on the counter in my kitchen is a masticating Hurom. Whatever brand or type you choose, you will get to know it intimately during the Cleanse, so be sure to read the instructions and to treat it well.

Blenders

When it comes to blenders, you face a similar choice between cheap and expensive. You can pick up a slower, less powerful Magic Bullet for $30; a high-speed, high-power Vitamix for $600; and everything in between.

The advantages of a high-powered blender are:

- They can blend nuts and seeds raw, without your having to soak them first.
- They can handle tougher vegetables like beets and carrots.
- They can handle sticky substances like tahini.
- They make super-smooth smoothies and soups.
- You can make smaller batches.

The blender on my counter is a Vitamix, but you will do fine with a NutriBullet, too. Again, it's up to you and what you're comfortable with.

On the Cleanse, you will use your equipment *a lot* and will get your money's worth regardless. Keep it simple. Do not stress about it. Just get what you need, and we can move right along!

In the next chapter, I'll go over two final components of the Cleanse—exercises for the body and the mind.

Nonessential (but Really Useful) Supplies

Just a few optional items to gather or take out of storage:

Portable BPA-free plastic or glass containers. I would recommend investing in a few good-quality containers that you can store and transport your meals in. Screw-on lids are a plus if you take your meals to work with you. The last thing you need during the Cleanse is a green soup spilled in your bag! Being a keen recycler, I love to use old coconut oil jars to store my juices and smoothies, and the really big mason jars for soups.

A portable cooler. An insulated zip bag with an ice pack is really useful for keeping meals cool in transport. It doesn't need to be expensive or fancy.

A quality vegetable peeler and good knives. You're going to be prepping a lot of vegetables, so it's smart to make the job as quick and easy as possible with a sharp-but-safe peeler and knives. If you have access to organic foods, you don't have to worry about peeling before juicing. But otherwise, you'll need proper blades for all those carrots and beets.

CHAPTER 10

EXERCISE ON THE ARC

On the ARC, there is an exercise component, but it's not as bad as you might fear. If anything, I want to make sure you're not *over*exercising on the Cleanse. If you were to go too hard, you'd put your body under stress, which is the last thing you want to do. The aim is to expel toxins, mobilize stagnant lymph, gently speed up metabolism, and deliver lots of lovely oxygen all over the place.

Everyone comes into the Cleanse at different exercise levels, and I'm sure you will find the right pace for yours. For example, if you are a never-exercise person, all you really need to do is take a 15- to 30-minute walk every day to elevate your heart rate slightly and increase oxygen intake. Previous clients who have chosen to take it easy and rest during the Cleanse did fine with light strolls or bike rides. On the other end of the spectrum, I've had clients who were enthusiastic gymgoers or elite athletes who felt great from Day One and carried on their demanding routine as normal throughout. If you're a seasoned exerciser, you can trust yourself and your instincts as to what you are able to do and handle. For the large swath in the middle between never-exercisers and dedicated athletes, I'd like you to try a few different types of exercise that will help you make the most of the Cleanse.

REBOUNDING

The ideal form of exercise on the Cleanse is rebounding, otherwise known as jumping up and down on a mini-trampoline. Like juicers and blenders, mini-tramps can be purchased for next to nothing (less than $50) or a fortune (close to $600). Clients of mine who got the $50 units were quite satisfied with them.

As for what to do on a mini-tramp once you have one, you can search online for videos of "rebounder workouts" and find dozens at every skill level. Or you can just hop on the mini-tramp and bounce up and down for 10 minutes with your feet barely leaving the mat. This minimum-impact rebounding is called "health bounce." All you're doing is letting momentum take your body up and down, up and down. It's easy and fun, and absolutely fantastic to do during the Cleanse.

Rebounding is probably the most detoxifying exercise possible. It gets the heart going and brings oxygen in. But more important and unique, it is one of the only movements you can do that actively mobilizes your lymphatic system. Baby hops on a little trampoline get your lymph circulating, which boosts the immune system thanks to the increase in white blood cell activity. Unlike your blood circulation system that is mobilized by a pump (the heart), the lymphatic circulation system is composed of one-way-flowing rivers and does not have a central pump. It opens up to allow greater volume of flow during changes of gravitational pull or g-force. When you land on the tramp and then bounce up, you are changing g-force over and over again, causing a surge of lymph to flow at a faster pace. As it flows, it sweeps up toxins, which will be moved to the kidneys and expelled in urine. The healthier the lymphatic drainage, the more toxins are cleansed. You will be ridding the body of pouches of stagnant, stuck lymph (the primary cause of cellulite) as you bounce away the toxins that cells release as a result of the Cleanse process.

What's more, rebounding is really easy on the joints, requires no experience, takes only a few minutes (10 minutes a day is good), and can be done rain or shine, all the while strengthening cells and building muscle fibers.

If you can't rebound due to such conditions as balance impairment from neuropathy or Ménière's disease, you can get the same g-force lymph benefits by sitting on a fitness ball with both feet planted on the floor.

Walking/Running

Moving is a must on the Cleanse, 15 to 30 minutes a day. Ultimately, you'll upgrade a daily walk into a speed walk, then a jog, and then a run, but start slow. If you aren't accustomed to running or jogging, please don't start on the

Cleanse! You'll put undue stress on your system, which alters your hormonal balance counterproductively.

If you do run a bit, and don't want to overtax your body, find a pace that works for the Cleanse and when you can, push yourself harder. It's actually very important that you exercise the right way on the Cleanse to stay alkaline.

What do I mean by that? Well, have you ever finished a run and felt sick and light-headed? Or have you finished a run and really needed a sugar hit? In both cases, you were exercising anaerobically, or using glucose stored in your muscles for energy instead of using incoming oxygen. Anaerobic exercise for long periods is acidifying, not alkalizing. In other words, it is the opposite of what you want.

Your goal during the Cleanse is to eliminate acids, toxins, and stored visceral fat, while lowering inflammation. You will do all that by exercising aerobically, with walking or easy jogging. This kind of moderate-intensity workout is highly alkalizing, improves your fitness level, strengthens your heart, boosts your metabolism, increases red blood cell count, and eliminates toxins from your body through your skin (sweat) and breath (respiratory system). It also triggers your body to go to slow-burn fat storage for energy, instead of grabbing quick-access carbohydrates (sugars), as it does during intense, anaerobic exercise.

The bottom line is, if you find yourself panting or gasping for breath and your heart is beating out of your chest, you are using sugar (not fat) for energy, increasing inflammation and clinging to stored acids. If you are breathing normally enough to talk and your heart rate is elevated somewhat, you will be burning fat, reducing inflammation, and purging stored acids.

Depending on what mode of exercise you're in—anaerobic or aerobic—your body will use different muscle fibers and access a different, primary energy source. The switch occurs when you hit a certain number of heartbeats per minute (BPM), and your body automatically shifts from an aerobic (fat burning, alkalizing) to an anaerobic (sugar burning, acidizing) response.

I'd say 98 percent of my clients are interested in finding and staying in the fat-burning zone during exercise. This zone is not one-formula-fits-all. To find it, you have to calculate the ideal BPM for you. It's not a hard computation, although there are different formulas. I recommend the Stu Mittleman method.[7] Mittleman is an ultramarathon champion who set the world record for the 1,000-mile run, completing it in 11 days. He also holds the U.S. record for the 6-day race of 578 miles, or 96 miles per day—the equivalent of 3.7 marathons.

7   I found this formula in Mittleman's book *Slow Burn: Burn Fat Faster by Exercising Slower*. If you'd like to go deeper, I highly recommend reading it.

In 2000, he ran the entire width of the U.S. in 55 days at a rate of 52 miles per day. We can consider him to be somewhat of an authority on aerobic training and running! He's also a strong advocate of the alkaline lifestyle and has based his entire training regimen for these extreme events on exercising correctly to ensure his energy is derived from fat, not sugar.

His method for calculating your fat-burn zones is simple:

180 – [your age] = maximum heart rate for aerobic, fat-burning exercise

If your BPM goes over that number, you will automatically switch into sugar-burn mode. If you feel dizzy and queasy after a run, your maximum heart rate is too high and you are burning sugar.

A 50-year-old's maximum fat-burn heart rate is 130 BPM (180 – 50 = 130). A 20-year-old's max fat-burn heart rate is 150 BPM. And so on.

Now, it gets slightly more complicated from there. Ideal target fat-burn rates are then broken down into three levels. The lowest level of intensity is the "warm-up zone" (WUZ). The middle level is the "mostly aerobic pace" (MAP). The highest is the "most efficient pace" (MEP).

For the purposes of the Cleanse, I want you to concentrate your efforts on MAP, the middle zone. It's where peak fat burning occurs, and it's the most friendly for detoxing and flushing out your lymphatic system. MAP can be calculated with this formula:

Maximum heart rate (180 – [your age]) – 10 = MAP upper limit

MAP upper limit – 10 = MAP lower limit

Using myself as an example, my maximum heart rate for fat burn is 143 (anything higher would be anaerobic), calculated as: 180 – 37 (my age) = 143.

To find my MAP *upper* limit, the equation is:

143 – 10 = 133.

To calculate my MAP *lower* limit, the equation is:

133 – 10 = 123.

So, when I run, I try to keep my heart rate between 133 and 123. If I pushed myself higher and went over my MAP upper limit, I'd be in MEP territory, which is absolutely fine, but it's not as ideal for fat burning. If I dipped *below* my MAP lower limit (from 123 to 113), I'd fall into WUZ for warming up (or cooling down).

For a 50-year-old, the numbers look like this:

180 – 50 = 130 BPM = maximum heart rate for fat burn = MEP upper limit

130 – 10 = 120 BPM = MEP lower limit = MAP upper limit

120 – 10 = 110 BPM = MAP lower limit = WUZ upper limit

110 – 10 = 100 BPM = WUZ lower limit

You might hit your MAP zone with brisk walking. You might have to intersperse walking with running (or vice versa). The good news is, once you've become an accomplished runner (running regularly for six months), it'll take more speed to get your heart going, and you can add 5 or 10 BPM to each zone.

Obviously, the best way to know your heart rate is to wear a wrist monitor like a Fitbit, Jawbone, or Apple Watch. You can download a free heart-rate app for any smartphone, but it won't give a continuous readout. I strongly urge you to invest in a wrist monitor. It's up there with a juicer as one of the most important investments you will ever make.

Are You in the Fat-Burn Zone?

YES

- You can talk normally without being short of breath.
- Your vision is clear.
- You have heightened senses of smell and sight.
- You are in a steady, comfortable rhythm.
- You would rate your level of intensity between four and seven.

NO

- You are short of breath, especially when talking.
- You feel dizzy or nauseated.
- You feel uncomfortable.
- You can't wait to finish.
- You would rate your level of intensity at above seven.

YOGA

I would *love* for you to do or try yoga during the Cleanse.

Even if you're not an experienced yogi, please try a few easy poses or take a beginner class and get your body stretching. Yoga is a huge support for your body as you detox. All that stretching, bending, and getting your head below your heart gets your lymph moving and brings oxygen to every cell. It's called a "moving meditation," and known to reduce stress, which is therefore balancing (literally) and anti-inflammatory.

So that's it! Some bouncing, walking, and stretching. Nothing crazy, nothing strenuous, and nothing to be scared of. Let your body be your guide about pace and frequency. The Cleanse isn't the right time to kick off a whole new regimen. Just make sure you get moving in some way, every day.

ARC Exercise Do's

The ARC is all about positivity—in food, fitness, and attitude. Just "do" your best, and *do not* worry if you miss a workout!

DO exercise in the morning, before your day officially begins. This tip comes from personal experience. I've been a runner for years, and I have found that unless I run as soon as I get up, I won't do it regularly. If I leave it until the afternoon, I'll find any excuse not to go (e.g., it's too late, I'm too busy, I'll go harder tomorrow). The key to success is to get into the habit of getting up, putting on your sneakers, and hitting the road before you brain is fully awake! (Oh, make sure you put on clothes, too!)

DO focus on time, not distance. The idea is to stay in your fat-burning zone for a certain amount of time. For one person, that might mean running seven-minute miles for an hour. For another, it might mean walking 15-minute miles for half an hour. Let your BPMs and stamina decide how intense and how long you exercise. No matter what your current level of fitness might be, you are working at a pace that is perfect *for you*, so do not go by a predetermined regimen you read online that was set by somebody else.

DO listen to your heart and stay in the right zone. Some may need to speed up a bit. Some exercise regulars will need to slow down. If you stay in the zone, you will burn fat, build strong muscles, and improve speed and endurance. After only a few short weeks of training in the right zones at the right speed, your aerobic capacity will very quickly increase. It will happen surprisingly fast, so don't feel like you are taking a step backward by slowing down for a while. It won't be long before you are back up to your previous speed, but you will find your heart rate staying low and feeling like you can run forever.

NON-SWEATY EXERCISES

Another exercise I'd like you to do on the Cleanse does not involve sneakers or sports bras. **I'd like you to do some breathing exercises.**

Along with your kidneys, liver, and skin, your lungs are detoxifying organs, too. You exhale waste with every breath, and, unfortunately, most of us are not making the most of our lungs. Shallow breathing into the chest only uses the lower part of the diaphragm, leaving the upper part inactive and collapsed. If you don't inhale into every part of your lungs, you're more prone to stress and negative emotions. (There's a reason why people say, "Just take a deep breath" to calm down, and why smokers relax as soon as they take that first deep lungful of smoke.)

In purely mechanical terms, when lobes of the lungs are chronically under-inflated, they gather a buildup of slimy mucus. The mucus irritates the cells of the lungs, causing an acid environment of irritation and inflammation. Mucus impairs the organ's self-cleaning system, tiny hairlike cilia that serve as lung sweepers. If these cilia are caked down in mucus, they can't clear germs and bacteria. (FYI: Smoke basically deadens cilia, and over time, the only way to get rid of mucus is what's called "smoker's cough.")

If you take deep, slow, directed, focused breaths to inflate the lower part of the lungs (the "belly" if you will), you can help your lungs stay clear and healthy, supporting them in their job of exhaling CO_2 and clearing microscopic irritants. It's simple, straightforward, *free*, and one of the best things you can do for your body.

Some of the benefits of taking level, deep, cleansing breaths include:

- **Stress reduction.** Those with stress and anxiety issues tend to take short, shallow breaths. Conversely, long, deep breathers report better control of their stress and anxiety.

- **Depression.** Research has found that deep, diaphragmatic breathing helps people suffering from depression.

- **Pain relief.** Deep breathing releases endorphins—natural painkillers—into your system. The next time that you have a headache, stomachache, or any other pains, imagine breathing into the place it hurts.

- **Asthma relief.** Deep breathing strengthens the lungs and the core, which helps asthmatics control their symptoms.

- **More energy.** Shallow breathing leads to inadequate oxygenation of the blood and fatigue.

- **Lymphatic cleansing.** Deep breathing can act as a kind of pump for the lymphatic system, cleansing and detoxifying your body.

You might be thinking, *Breathing is something you do all day long. It's not something I'm going to be able to stop and think about.*

But you can . . . if you link it to something you already do and create a new habit, like hydration or walking. On the ARC, I've built breathing exercises into your daily schedule, so that you will remember to do them. They're part of the Cleanse's structure, so it's impossible for you to forget about them. Before long, you'll feel strange if you *don't* do them.

When I first started consistently practicing breathing exercises, I experienced an immediate, noticeable effect. My energy increase was incredible, as well as mental clarity, especially in the afternoon when I was starting to lag. I became so much more effective and got so much more done! The first few days required some serious alarm reminders and Post-it Notes, but in no time, the exercises became as habitual as washing my face and brushing my teeth. I'd have my morning oils and automatically know that it was also time to practice deep breathing.

Breathing Exercise #1: Basic Deep Breathing

Three simple steps:

1. Lie flat on your back.

2. Put your hands gently on your belly at the bottom of your ribs with your fingertips just touching each other.

3. Take a slow, deep breath, letting your belly rise slightly, which will separate your fingertips.

Breathing with your belly may feel unnatural at first, so repeat this 30 times or until breathing with your chest feels like an unnatural action. When you breathe deeply into your belly, the diaphragm creates a suction, drawing air up into the lungs. This fills the bloodstream with wonderful acid-fighting oxygen and expels carbon dioxide, cleansing the body of the acid wastes and their harmful by-products.

Breathing Exercise #2: The Lymphatic Cleanse

I call this "power breathing," and it's one of the best, most effective exercises you can do for free, every day, in five minutes. It is also remarkably simple. I learned the lymphatic cleanse exercise from Tony Robbins.[8] He swears by it, and I'm not going to argue with his energy levels!

It's all about inhaling, holding, and exhaling, in a particular rhythm.

1. Inhale for one count

2. Hold for four counts

3. Exhale for two counts

The golden ratio is one-four-two. If you prefer to inhale for two counts, then hold for eight and exhale for four. I recommend going through the cycle 10 times, at least once a day, during the Cleanse, but ideally twice (right after you wake up and before you go to sleep, for example). As far as the Cleanse goes, I've taken the liberty of adding these exercises to your daily schedule, but there's no time like *now* to give them a go and incorporate them into your life before you start.

Which is exactly what comes next: the week before the Cleanse. The countdown begins in the next chapter. We've spent 10 chapters covering the nuts and bolts of how and why the Alkaline Reset Cleanse works. We've worn the operations manager hat. You now know why people fall out of balance, and the impact the ARC will have on your Five Master Systems. I've explained why I've chosen the foods you'll be eating (and why you need to cut out others). We've gone over the supplements and equipment you'll need, the aerobic and breathing exercises you'll need to do. Big picture? You have a perfect, 10,000-foot aerial view of the ARC.

---

8   Another great technique from *Unlimited Power.*

Next, we'll be zooming in on the small details of what you'll actually be doing each day.

This is where the rubber hits the road.

Everyone, start your engines (and blenders)!

PART III

LET'S
DO IT!

CHAPTER 11

THE SEVEN DAYS BEFORE THE CLEANSE

Priming your body for your Cleanse is a smart move. If you take a few simple steps in the seven days *before* your Cleanse, it will be an easier, more powerful process and, ultimately, a more enjoyable experience. Some basic prep work will give you more energy during the ARC and reduce the risk of detox symptoms. Look, you prepare for most things in life, for a new job or a trip abroad. You prepare for a run by warming up. The week before the Cleanse is just another way to warm up.

In this case, it's a hell of warm-up! It's common for people to reach some of their Cleanse goals during the seven days before. When you focus your attention on just a few simple habits that help your body restore balance, your health lifts so rapidly, it's truly amazing.

By the end of the "before" stage, you will have reduced cravings for foods and drinks that cause detox symptoms (caffeine-withdrawal headaches, for example), and you will have made giant strides toward scrubbing your liver, kidneys, and digestive system. Clean, detoxed organs mean your body is ready and eager to receive and make excellent use of the ultra-nourishment to come from the juices, soups, and smoothies.

Now, I should say that prep week is *not* mission critical. If you need to do the Cleanse *immediately, today,* then you could just dive into it now. But if you come in prepared—logistically and physiologically—you will get so much more out of it. Taking a week beforehand to test recipes, practice exercises, do your shopping, and start taking certain supplements will compound your positive results. If you can, follow these steps for *more* than seven days before, and you'll be shocked how strong, vital, and ready you feel to take on the world!

Big-Picture Planning

Generally, when it comes to getting from where you are now with your health to where you want to be, planning is *everything.* I have done pretty much all of the planning for you, including a full "seven days before" meal plan and shopping lists, available for free at rossbridgeford.com/arc. In this book, I've included a looser-form version of the meal plans. Beyond food, there are a few things to take care of to make your journey as effortless and enjoyable as possible.

Prep Step #1: Commit to a Saturday Start Date

There will never be a *perfect* week to do the ARC. Any seven-day period will have some event or conflict that could present a challenge. However, there are better weeks (and weekends) than others. Look ahead in your calendar at the next 90 days (not further out than that; things can easily change and you might run the risk of postponing your Cleanse even further into the future).

I highly recommend you start on a Saturday. *This is important.* This gives you the whole weekend, Saturday and Sunday, to get used to the process, and to go through any detox symptoms you might have. Come Monday, at the start of the workweek, you'll be an old pro at juicing, and any fatigue or aches and pains will be behind you. Of course, if you don't work or you work from home or your workweek begins on a Wednesday, adjust your start day accordingly so you basically have two "free days" to get into the swing of it before you resume your responsibilities in full. You also can spend the weekend (or whichever free days you choose) to make some of the soup recipes for the week ahead and put them in the freezer. Juices and smoothies should be consumed within a day of making them (ideally, within 12 hours), but you can get a jump on Monday by preparing the ingredients on Sunday.

Okay, so check your calendar right now. What one-week stretch in the next three months looks the emptiest right now? Can you reschedule some plans to make it even better? If you see a good week, block it out now. Commit to it.

Between now and then, you can start the "before" protocol, even if your start date is a few weeks away. Might as well!

Prep Step #2: Order Supplements

As soon as you have your Cleanse start date, order your supplements. You'd be surprised how long it can take for certain ones to arrive. If any supplement has not arrived by your start date, *do not use this as an excuse to delay*. On the ARC, you will be getting a huge amount of nourishment, and you don't really need to have any supplements to get fabulous results.

Prep Step #3: Buy or Borrow Equipment

If you don't have a blender or juicer, order online, borrow, or pick one up ASAP. Without these two items, you cannot do the Cleanse. In fact, you might as well go buy them today in a store (is shopping in person still a thing?) to guarantee that you have no reason to put things off.

Once you have an official start date, your supplements, and your equipment, you have pretty much done all the planning you need to do. I've taken care of all the rest. To make this as simple and easy as possible, I have broken down each day of the prep week and the Cleanse itself for you. Each day is as important as the next, and if you follow these steps, you *will* experience success. All you need to do now is follow along and get the radiant health it brings!

Day-By-Day: The Seven Days BEFORE the Cleanse

You can do the before phase for as long as you like. You don't have to limit it to seven days! If your Cleanse date is scheduled for a month from now and you start the prep now, so much the better!

DAY ONE

Saturday (or Your "Saturday")

Set Goals and Get Excited!

Today is all about feeling the excitement and the natural buzz you get when you do something amazing for yourself. That sense of accomplishment will give you a confidence boost, and you can take that momentum forward. By the end of today, I want you to feel empowered!

One way to feel that surge is by setting goals for your health—not just about what you hope to get out of the ARC, but beyond. Just around the corner, you'll have new energy and a new body. What will you do with them? Day One of prep week is the perfect time to set your biggest, wildest health goals and start making them a reality.

I believe setting goals is one of the most powerful things you can do to transform your life. Of course, doing just that can be overwhelming (we all want to do and be so many things!). The key is simplicity and understanding. Along with understanding what your goals are, you have to be clear on why you have them. If the *what* and *why* are solid in your mind, you'll be far more likely to finish the Cleanse, and take your success forward.

Your Goal-Setting Plan

This approach is as simple as it gets, which is one of the reasons it works:

- Write down your goals. Specifically, top the list with your immediate goals for the Cleanse itself, and then keep going with your long-term health goals for the rest of your life. You might write something like, "I have the goal of completing the Cleanse and making the most of it, and I hope to eat healthy and be active from now on."

- Write down what your life will be like if you reach those goals, for example, "If I stick to the Cleanse and a healthy lifestyle, I'll live a long, disease-free, energized life."

- Then, put down what your life would be like if you *don't* reach those goals, as in, "If I don't stick with a healthy lifestyle, I might wind up sick and old before my time with a poor quality of life."

- Finally, make a list of the people you're doing this for besides yourself—your partner, kids, parents, or friends. Link your goals to something outside of yourself to access the full power of goal setting.

If you reread (ideally, rewrite) your goals each night before you go to sleep, you will harness the incredible power of clarity.

Day One Meal Plan

Upon Waking: Turmeric and Coconut Tea
Breakfast: Super-Nutrient Breakfast Bowl
Snack: Antioxidant Green Smoothie
Lunch: The usual (whatever you'd usually have)
Snack: Easy Bliss Balls
Dinner: The usual

Since this is prep week, you don't have to follow the meal plan to the letter. But I'd like you to familiarize yourself with a couple of recipes that you'll be making during the ARC and to break in your blender. This menu gives you a huge hit of nourishment, helps you fall in love with healthy foods, and builds the foundation of great habits.

The day starts with creamy Turmeric and Coconut Tea—a warming, filling, soothing, comforting *yet powerfully alkaline and anti-inflammatory* hot beverage. It's one of my most popular recipes, and although it requires a tiny amount of prep, it will get easier every time. Some people report feeling a little queasy drinking a high dose of fats on an empty stomach (but only at first). If that happens to you, wipe out the nauseated feeling with a quick snack of any food you have at hand. If your diet has been unbalanced for a while, it might be a good idea to halve the fats in the recipe the first few times you make it.

TURMERIC AND COCONUT TEA

Makes 2 servings

Ingredients

1 tablespoon fresh root turmeric, grated
12 ounces filtered (preferably alkaline) water
¼ teaspoon garam masala

½ teaspoon ground cinnamon
1 tablespoon grass-fed butter
1 tablespoon coconut oil or MCT oil
Pinch of stevia to taste (optional)

Instructions

Grate the turmeric into a pan with the water, garam masala, and cinnamon. Simmer for 5 to 10 minutes.

Pour the contents of the pan into a blender (straining out the turmeric bits). Add the butter and oil and blend at high speed until foamy and creamy! Add a pinch of stevia, if desired, to taste.

For breakfast, I've included my Super-Nutrient Breakfast Bowl, a colorful, cooked, protein-rich, alkaline-rich treat of a brekkie. It takes 15 minutes to make, and it's a real gift for yourself—an antioxidant, alkalizing delicious start to the day!

SUPER-NUTRIENT BREAKFAST BOWL

Makes 2 servings

Ingredients

1 large sweet potato
2 tablespoons coconut oil, divided
2 garlic cloves, finely chopped
8 broccoli florets
2 large handfuls of beet greens or kale

4 large handfuls of baby spinach
1 large avocado, roughly chopped
1 tablespoon sunflower seeds
1 tablespoon chia seeds
Salt and cracked pepper to taste

Lemon & Tahini Alkaline Dressing

4 tablespoons tahini (homemade or purchased)
4 tablespoons filtered water
2 tablespoons flax or olive oil

Juice of 1 lemon
2 teaspoons grated fresh gingerroot
Himalayan salt and cracked black pepper to taste

Instructions

Preheat the oven to 400°F (200°C). While the oven is heating, wash the sweet potato and slice thinly (more like a chip than a wedge). Put the slices on the baking sheet, coat them with 1 tablespoon of the coconut oil, and season with salt and pepper. Toss until evenly coated. Bake for 15 to 20 minutes until crisp (keep an eye on these; they can go from perfect to burnt in a minute).

While the potatoes are cooking, make the dressing. Combine all the dressing ingredients in a blender or food processor and blend until smooth.

Prepare the veggies. Gently heat the remaining 1 tablespoon coconut oil in a large pan over medium heat. Add the garlic and cook for 1 minute. Then add the broccoli, beet greens, and spinach. Warm through for 4 or 5 minutes until the greens are wilted and the broccoli is al dente.

Remove the potatoes from the oven and pat down with a paper towel. Line the bowls (one for now, one in a container to refrigerate and save for later) with the potatoes, then add the veggies and the avocado, sprinkle with the seeds, and top with the dressing. Season to taste with salt and pepper.

Next, a midmorning snack. Get ready to make your first smoothie. I call it my Antioxidant Green Smoothie. The first two recipes were heavy on the alkalinity and anti-inflammatories. This smoothie hits the third of the Triple As: antioxidants! This concoction will fill you up for hours. I like to have it after a workout or for breakfast, and it keeps me going for ages.

ANTIOXIDANT GREEN SMOOTHIE

Makes 2 servings

Ingredients

1 avocado
1 cucumber
Juice of ½ lemon
1 handful of kale
1 handful of spinach

2 heads of broccoli
1 tomato
1 handful of lettuce
½ garlic clove
Filtered water

Instructions

Place the avocado, cucumber, and lemon juice in a blender and process to form a mushy paste, then start adding the other ingredients until everything is evenly blended.

Relax and have a "normal" lunch—and dinner for that matter—of whatever you like. You can be healthy, unhealthy, it's totally up to you. Think of prep week as a free-for-all. For a midafternoon snack, make a batch of my wildly popular Easy Bliss Balls. These will last for a few days in the fridge; they're great to have whenever a "snack attack" strikes.

EASY BLISS BALLS

Makes 2 servings

Ingredients

4 Medjool dates
¼ cup almonds
1 cup almond meal
⅓ cup pistachios, divided

½ cup shredded coconut
⅓ cup coconut oil
⅓ cup cacao powder
1 tablespoon chia seeds

Instructions

Remove the seeds from the dates. Soften the dates and the 1/4 cup of almonds in hot water for an hour. Ideally, you'd soak the almonds for 4 hours, but an hour is fine. (If you have a high-speed blender or food processor, no softening is needed.)

Blend together the dates, almonds, almond meal, half the pistachios, the shredded coconut, coconut oil, cacao, and chia seeds.

Transfer the mixture to a bowl and let stand for a few minutes to allow the chia to soften and expand.

Smash the remaining pistachios. Roll the date mixture into small balls and then roll them in the crushed pistachios to coat.

Day One Checklist

- Familiarize yourself with the foods and meals coming up. Are there any foods you're allergic or intolerant to? Swap these for similar ingredients.

- Look ahead in your calendar. Are there any events that could make it difficult to stick to the plan? Sort out a Plan B to get around these hurdles. Preparation and awareness are the key to making things easy.

- Write out your goals! Put pen and paper next to your bed so you can rewrite them before sleep or as soon as you wake up.

DAY TWO
Sunday (or Your "Sunday")

Build on Positive Momentum

Today I want you to build on the success of yesterday. Sometimes, because they've had a successful Day One, people relax *too much* on Day Two. So focus and stay present in your goals. I'd also like you to practice your preprep skills and get some of tomorrow's hard work out of the way. For most of you, Day Three will be on a Monday, your first day back at work and, most likely, out of the house. You'll have to do double the cooking on Sunday to make enough to bring to the office on Monday for your lunch and snacks. Cooking on Sunday for Monday is a habit that will transform your life.

Speaking of habits, give some attention to perhaps the most powerful health habit you can make: your water consumption. Many people who come to me for help with health issues have been chronically dehydrated for years. Don't be one of those people! It's a free and easy fix; it just takes forming a new small habit.

Hydration *has* to become an important part of your life from now on! Being dehydrated is damaging to practically every area, system, and process in your body. It creates massive imbalance, inflammation, digestive clogging, and acidity. It takes two minutes per day to drink enough water. There are really no excuses!

If you have less than a liter of water per day—especially if you drink coffee, regular tea, or alcohol daily—you *really* need to prime your body for the Cleanse by getting a minimum of two liters of water per day right now, building up to three by Day One of the during stage. Getting up to three liters by Day Five of prep week would be fantastic, with two being your minimum target. If you do that, hydration will do a lot of the early heavy lifting of the Cleanse, allowing the nutrients to go straight to work.

Your Hydration Plan

It's all about awareness! Ask yourself:

- What is my daily water intake (water, herbal teas, green juices) now?

- What is my intake of diuretic, a.k.a. dehydrating liquids (coffee, alcohol, black tea, soda)?

- What is my hydration goal by Day Five of the before week?

- What is my hydration goal by Day One of the during week?
- What is my hydration goal for the rest of my life?

Commit to counting your water intake every day. Start writing it down, use an app like Daily Water, or manually set alarms on your phone to remind you to drink.

Day Two Meal Plan

Upon Waking: Digestive Tea
Breakfast: The usual
Snack: Easy Bliss Balls
Lunch: The usual
Snack: Celery and Almond Butter Boats
Dinner: Lentil and Quinoa Stew

Today's meal plan is really simple. You already have the Bliss Balls premade from yesterday, and you'll have a "normal" breakfast and lunch. Start the day with my Digestive Tea, a simple, super-clean and fresh-tasting anti-inflammatory.

DIGESTIVE TEA

Makes 2 servings

Ingredients

2 cups filtered water
2 teaspoons fennel seeds

2 inches fresh gingerroot, peeled and chopped or thinly sliced
1 tablespoon peppermint leaf or regular mint

Instructions

Add the water, fennel, ginger, and mint to a pot.
Bring to a boil, then lower the heat to a very gentle simmer. After 5 minutes, turn off the heat and steep the tea for 5 to 10 minutes.
Serve warm.

For an afternoon snack, you'll have one of my favorite alkaline treats, a Celery and Almond Butter Boat, legendary for how fast and easy it is to make and how it keeps you going!

CELERY AND ALMOND BUTTER BOAT

Makes 2 servings

Ingredients

1 celery stick
Almond butter (or any nut butter except peanut)

Instructions

Chop the celery stick into 2-inch pieces, then spread the almond butter liberally down the middle. Easy!

Dinner tonight (and lunch tomorrow) is Lentil and Quinoa Stew, hearty and delicious, super-alkaline, and anti-inflammatory. One of the tricks of food preparation is to make more than you need. If you have the equipment out, the vegetables ready, and the time put aside to cook, why not make a little more for later? If you wind up with too much for dinner and lunch, put it in a freezer bag and mark it with the date. You can eat it anytime within three months.

LENTIL AND QUINOA STEW

Makes 2 servings

Ingredients

1 cup dry lentils
5 cups filtered water, divided
1 tablespoon coconut oil
1 yellow onion, diced
3 carrots, diced
3 celery stalks, sliced
4 garlic cloves, crushed
1 ½ teaspoons ground cumin

½ teaspoon ground ginger
½ teaspoon ground turmeric
2 teaspoons salt, plus more to taste
½ cup dry quinoa
2 cups chopped kale, tough stems removed
One 12-ounce can chopped tomatoes or 6 fresh tomatoes

Instructions

Put the lentils in a pot and cover with 2 cups of filtered water. Bring to a boil, then reduce the heat to a simmer. Cover and cook until the liquid is gone and the lentils are tender (check regularly). This will take approximately 30 minutes.

When the lentils are done, set them aside in a bowl. Wipe down the pan and warm the coconut oil in it. Sauté the onions, carrots, and celery for 5 or 6 minutes. Then stir in the spices and salt.

Stir in the quinoa, remaining water, kale, and chopped tomatoes (if using fresh, blend first) and bring to a boil.

Lower the heat and cook until the quinoa has uncoiled and is tender, about 12 minutes. Add in the lentils and stir until evenly mixed.

Day Two Checklist

- Make your hydration plan! Planning and mental preparation is key to making this happen. Hydration can easily slip by unless you consciously make a plan and put in the effort. After a few days it will become an effortless habit, but for the first few days or a week, it will need focus.

- Rewrite your goals.

- Order any supplements you might need for the during phase.

- Get out your juicer and make sure it's in full working order!

DAY THREE
Welcome to the Workweek

Fix a Major Nutrient Deficiency

Day Three of the before week is a tricky one. It's the first *real* hurdle because, if you're like most people, you're out of the house and on the go. Ninety percent of the time, outside-the-house snacks are acidic and inflammatory (they don't sell Bliss Balls at the corner store). It's so important today to be prepared and to have your goals on the forefront of your mind. Think ahead: Can you bring a smoothie or soup to work with you? Is there a juice bar nearby that makes organic green drinks and smoothies? Now is the time to look around for options and figure out your plan for transporting your snacks, soups, and smoothies to work with you.

Most people are chronically deficient in healthy fats—omega 3 (we tend to get enough omega 6 and 9; often too much of them) and saturated fat from coconuts. Many wrongly believe all fats are unhealthy and try to avoid them.

The truth is, good fats heal, repair, and restore your body, speed your metabolism, reduce inflammation, support weight loss, lower LDL cholesterol, increase HDL cholesterol, and protect and fortify the brain. What substances *do* make you gain weight? Sugar, refined foods, fast foods, toxic foods, additives, chemicals and preservatives, gluten, and cheap junk food. Starting today, to help prevent hunger between meals and keep your blood sugar balanced, you will up your consumption of healthy fats.

Your Healthy Fats Plan

- Add three tablespoons of omega 3 per day.
- Add one tablespoon of coconut oil per day.

It takes less than a minute a day to swallow a few capsules, but that small action will instantly reduce inflammation, support your liver, and unclog your small intestine where the nutrient absorption takes place.

It's hard to get enough of these fats consistently from diet alone, especially omega 3, and particularly on the Cleanse, despite eating foods that are high in it like flaxseed, chia seed, beans, greens, and cabbage. Before and after the ARC, oily fish is not disqualified from your diet. But just to make sure you get enough every day, add these fats for a huge uplift in your health and energy, for basically almost no work required.

Day Three Meal Plan

Upon Waking: Turmeric and Coconut Tea
Breakfast: Simple Alkaline Oats
Snack: Celery and Almond Butter Boats
Lunch: Leftover stew from yesterday
Snack: Easy Bliss Balls
Dinner: The usual

Today your main assignment is to make sure you don't skip an alkaline breakfast! Start with the Turmeric and Coconut Tea and follow up with Simple Alkaline Oats. These two recipes together give you all three Triple As, as well as a healthy hit of fats, fiber, and protein. You will be full for hours. Oats, by the way, are gluten-free, and make it quick, simple, and easy to tick the alkaline box at breakfast.

SIMPLE ALKALINE OATS

Makes 2 servings

Ingredients

½ to 1 cup oats (depending on how hungry you are)
1 to 2 cups filtered water (depending on how many oats you prepare)
1 teaspoon chia seeds

A splash of nut milk
1 teaspoon coconut oil
1 teaspoon cinnamon
A dollop of coconut or nondairy yogurt
1 handful of mixed nuts and seeds
Berries of your choice, optional

Instructions

Bring the oats and *water* (not milk!) to a simmer in a pan, then add the chia seeds. Cook until the mixture is a touch too dry for your liking, then stir in a splash or 2 of the nut milk. (I love coconut milk, but any other nondairy milk is fine.)

Remove the oats from the heat and stir in the coconut oil, cinnamon, and a dollop of nondairy yogurt. Top with the nuts and seeds and then finish with blueberries or strawberries, if desired. (I recommend keeping your fructose intake down to 1 or 2 servings of in-season fruit per day.)

If you do get a little hungry before lunch, snack on Celery and Almond Butter Boats (the ones you brought to work with you) to fill up on fiber, fats, and protein.

Go ahead and have your regular dinner—whatever you choose, it's up to you—but I *do* urge you to take your leftover Lentil and Quinoa Stew from yesterday to work for your lunch. If that's not possible, choose a healthy option today like a salad. Every positive decision you make for your body builds momentum going into the Cleanse.

Day Three Checklist

- Follow your hydration plan.

- Rewrite your goals.

- Starting today, add supplements with healthy fats. If you still don't have them, make a trip to the store today. Just about any grocery store will have organic coconut oil and omega-3 capsules. No excuses!

DAY FOUR

Work on an Acid Addiction.

You've reached the halfway point of the before phase and maybe you're starting to feel some benefits already. I'm sure you're full of positivity and anticipation about the during phase, the real deal of the ARC, coming up in just a few more days. There's still some priming to do, though. For the next four days, you're going to ramp up your alkaline meals and get your body ready for the big week ahead.

Today's focus is on transitioning away from acids. So far, you've been upping your alkaline, and it's been pretty easy. Just add water, fats, and turmeric (so much turmeric!). Superb. But now it's going to get just a touch harder. Now a little tough love comes in.

You already know that the ARC is not only about upping the good stuff in your life, like Triple A foods, bouncing, and breathing. It's also about eliminating the bad stuff. You already know when you're consuming something that isn't alkaline or cleansing—coffee, chocolate, sugar, wine, ice cream, white bread, junk food. I need you to begin moving away from that stuff, starting now.

In an ideal world, you'd cut all the acid-forming foods and substances before the Cleanse, so that you're 100 percent over your detox symptoms and cravings on Day One of the during stage. But I know that's not entirely realistic, nor what you're inclined to do in the before stage. It's daunting to be so strict, so suddenly. Only a few days ago, it's possible you were having coffee, bagels, and bacon for breakfast every day. And now, you're having turmeric tea and almond milk oatmeal. You're already making huge changes! I'm not going to ask you to give up *everything* acidic until you start the Cleanse itself. But you'll do yourself a huge favor by starting to cut down as much as you can now.

View the week before as a runway, where you get up to speed before you take off into the Cleanse. It's an opportunity to lower your intake, one day at a time, one substance at a time, before you hit altitude on Saturday (or whichever day you will start the ARC). It'll be easier for you then, and honestly, cutting back won't be as hard as you think it will be now. All you need (and this will shock you, coming from me) . . . *is a plan.*

Your Acid Elimination Plan

The easiest way to cut back is to reduce in increments. For instance, if you're currently having three cups of coffee a day, tomorrow, make it two cups. The day after tomorrow, make it one and a half. The day after that, one cup, and so on, until coffee is replaced by one of the turmeric teas.

If you're used to putting sugar and syrups in your lattes, perhaps tomorrow you could have the latte with just sugar. The day after that, a latte with no sugar. The day after that, a medium unsweetened latte instead of a large. Then a small instead of a medium. You get it. Wean yourself.

The same goes for wine and beer, too. Gently reduce the number of glasses until all alcohol is replaced with filtered water. And bread: If you usually have a whole bagel a day, can you make it a half tomorrow and a quarter the day after? If you're having a lot of sugar, how can you taper it down so that you're sugar free for the 24 hours before the Cleanse?

It helps to write down your daily goals for tapering off sugar, gluten, coffee, regular tea, alcohol, and processed foods. Between today and Saturday, what increments of acid foods and drinks will you have with the aim of halving or quartering the amounts down to zero?

This does bring up the point of not being aware of how much of a substance you're consuming. There are hidden chemicals in a lot of foods, even allegedly "healthy" ones. Assume anything in a wrapper has chemicals and additives—and sugars!

In my experience, most people's sugar intake is coming from just a small number of big offenders. By working out what your biggest sources of sugar are, you can easily swap these for sugar-free alternatives and get your sugar intake down by 80 percent overnight.

First, write down everything you've had to eat and drink over the past three days.

Next, go to nutritiondata.self.com, plug in your info, and you'll see the total sugars in each food, meal, and ingredient. Usually the 80/20 rule applies; you'll probably see that 80 percent of your sugar intake is coming from 20 percent of the foods and drinks you're having.

Then, cut out the top offenders, and replace them with sugar-free or low-sugar, nutrient-dense alternatives. (Watch out for sugar substitutes, though; they are just as acidic, inflammatory, and oxidizing as the real thing.) For example, if your store-bought jar of tomato sauce is packed with sugar, replace it with a can of crushed San Marzano tomatoes. Heat some chopped garlic and coconut oil in a pan, add the tomatoes, some sea salt, some basil. It's got just as much flavor as the stuff in a jar with zero added sugar, and it's less expensive.

There is always a healthier way. It might take a little more effort, but you can find it and will benefit from it.

Replacing Bad with Good: The Swish Method

No, this is not about how to sink a basketball.

Swish is a method of neurolinguistic programming (like self-hypnosis) that can help you change anything in your life—any response, reaction, craving, addiction, emotion, fear, and frustration. It's fast, and powerful, and you can do it right now.

The basic idea behind Swish (a.k.a. Visual Swish) is to replace one image (addiction, thought, emotion, behavior) with a more useful, positive one. It's telling the brain, "Don't do that, do this!" so that, over time, your old unproductive thought or behavior is automatically switched to the better one.

To try it, **pick one thing you want to change**. For example, what food or drink do you want to eliminate before the Cleanse? Many people really hate to give up coffee, so let's go with that.

The next step is to **identify the cue or trigger.** Perhaps it's the idea of sitting down for breakfast with your mug or the aroma of coffee brewing. Maybe it's walking by Starbucks. What stimulus makes your brain think *coffee*? Make a list.

Once you know your triggers, **create your ideal response** to them. What response would you prefer your brain to have instead? How about a detailed image of you, happy, confident, free of addictions, and smiling as you walk down the street with a green juice in your hand? The idea is to train your brain to swap the coffee craving for something different, so every time you're triggered for the acid food, your mind brings up a happy alternative, not a replacement substance (green juice for coffee) or a negative message ("Don't drink coffee!"), but an ideal version of yourself, successful in every area of life.

Can you picture it? Good. Take it up another level. Close your eyes and add details about where you are and what you're wearing. If this makes you smile and feel good on the inside, you've got it! If not, keep adding and adjusting and brightening until it does. Picture it vividly. Don't just see it. Feel it, too. Memorize every detail, and congratulate yourself. You have created your ideal response.

Just for a minute, think about something completely off topic. Your pet, your garden, anything. You have to briefly reset your brain off the subject at hand to **break state**, or reset your brain back to normal thinking.

Now the magic happens. You are going to program your brain to automatically replace an old thought pattern or behavior with a new, awesome one whenever it receives a trigger or cue. Here goes:

Retrigger *coffee*. Picture a hot mug of it in your mind. Make that mug bigger and see every detail. See yourself drinking it.

Now see a small picture of your ideal response image (you, radiating energy, happiness, and success) and put it down in the bottom right-hand corner of that giant coffee cup image. Make it small, dark, a bit fuzzy.

And now, the Swish! Move the small ideal response image of you farther and farther into the background until it's a tiny dot. Some people like to imagine it is being pulled back on an elastic band or slingshot. Then, fire the new tiny image at full power, back toward you. As it comes hurtling toward you, getting brighter, bigger, and more powerful, send the old trigger image (that steaming mug) flying back in the opposite direction until it becomes darker, smaller, and less powerful.

Optional: Make an audible "swishhhh" sound while you do it!

After you've done this a couple of times and really feel the joy of your idealized response image, quickly break state and think of something unrelated.

Consider yourself swished.

To **embed the change**, or lock it in, repeat this Swish pattern 10 times. It won't take long and it is so worth the mental effort. The results will last you forever and make it dramatically easier to choose healthy.

Day Four Meal Plan

Upon Waking: Creamy Coconut, Turmeric, and Ginger Warmer
Breakfast: The usual
Snack: Piece of fruit (your choice)
Lunch: The usual
Snack: Turmeric Roasted Nuts
Dinner: Anti-Inflammatory Soup

Today we're increasing your intake of the powerful anti-inflammatory turmeric, giving you two to three servings a day to help your body set the wheels in motion to soothe your inflammation before we even start the during phase.

There are other amazing anti-inflammatory foods—ginger, garlic, bell pepper, beetroot—but turmeric is by far the strongest. Taking in one centimeter of fresh root turmeric and/or a teaspoon of powdered, organic turmeric every day will make a noticeable, significant impact on your life, health, and energy within days. So many in my ARC coaching program have seen dramatic improvements of their inflammation-based conditions—pain, swelling, arthritis symptoms, sleep problems—just from adding daily turmeric to their diet, which is why I'm asking you to add it to yours, too.

Start the day with comforting, delicious Creamy Coconut, Turmeric, and Ginger Warmer. Have Turmeric Roasted Nuts as a flavor-packed midafternoon snack. Then, for dinner, enjoy Anti-Inflammation Soup with turmeric and lentil. In one day, over three meals, you'll learn just how easy it is to sneak anti-inflammatories into your daily life—and just how tasty they can be.

CREAMY COCONUT, TURMERIC, AND GINGER WARMER

Makes 2 servings

Ingredients

1 inch fresh turmeric root
½ inch fresh gingerroot
1 cup full-fat coconut milk (don't worry, coconut milk fat doesn't make you fat)

2 teaspoons coconut oil
1 cup coconut water (or filtered water)
1 teaspoon cloves
1 vanilla pod, optional
A pinch of black pepper* (optional)

Note: Black pepper is reported to help absorption and bioavailabiliy of the curcumin in turmeric.

Instructions

Peel the turmeric and ginger and grate into a mortar.

Add the coconut oil and using the pestle, turn it into a beautiful orange-yellow paste.

Pour the coconut milk and water into a pan and spoon in the turmeric-ginger paste. Add the cloves and the vanilla pod. Add a pinch of black pepper, if desired.

Simmer for 4 to 5 minutes.

Serve warm, straining if you wish.

TURMERIC ROASTED NUTS

Makes 4 to 6 servings

Ingredients

2 teaspoons coconut oil, melted
1 teaspoon turmeric powder
¾ teaspoon chili powder (or more to taste)
½ teaspoon fine sea salt
A good pinch of cracked black pepper
2 cups raw cashews

Instructions

Preheat the oven to 350°F (180° C). Line a baking sheet with parchment paper.

Combine the coconut oil, turmeric, chili powder, salt, and pepper in a mixing bowl. Add the cashews and coat well with the spice mix. Have a taste and feel free to add a little more of whatever you need.

Spread out the mixture in an even layer on the baking sheet and place in the oven for 10 minutes. Halfway through, stir the nuts, then pop them back in for another 5 minutes or until they're beautifully golden.

Cool and serve. Once they reach room temperature, place any remaining nuts in an airtight glass jar. They'll keep well in the pantry for weeks.

ANTI-INFLAMMATORY SOUP

Makes 2 servings

Ingredients

4 carrots
1 inch fresh gingerroot
1 inch fresh turmeric root
1 tablespoon coconut oil
1 red onion
8 ounces pumpkin
1 sweet potato
4 tomatoes
½ red pepper

3 garlic cloves
1 teaspoon mustard seeds
1 cup organic low-sodium vegetable stock
1 cup dry lentils
1 cup coconut cream
1 handful of fresh cilantro, chopped
1 thinly sliced red chili pepper, optional

Optional Topping

½ cup cashews
2 tablespoons pumpkin seeds

Coconut oil, to taste
1 garlic clove, minced

Instructions

Peel the carrots, ginger, and turmeric. Roughly chop *all the vegetables and the tomatoes*. (A lot of chopping. It'll be worth it!)

Gently heat the coconut oil in a pan, then add the onion. Cook for 1 or 2 minutes, then add the turmeric, ginger, mustard seeds, and garlic. Be careful not to burn the garlic.

Add the carrot, pumpkin, sweet potato, red pepper, and tomatoes, and stir to coat the veggies in the oil. (You should be able to smell that delicious turmeric now.)

Add the stock, then add the lentils.

Turn down to a simmer for 15 minutes while the veggies soften and the lentils cook. Once everything has softened, add the coconut cream and cilantro.

Use an immersion blender and blend until smooth, or transfer the mixture to a blender in batches. If using a regular blender, allow the soup to vent or the steam will make the top explode and you'll have soup all over your walls and ceiling.

To make the optional topping (which I've found really nice for adding a delicious extra texture to the soup), smash up the cashews under a knife and cook with the pumpkin seeds in a little coconut oil with the minced garlic until it's warmed through and slightly browned.

Serve the soup in bowls with a sprig of cilantro, a drizzle of coconut cream, and the cashew topping (plus the chili pepper, if using) and enjoy!

Day Four Checklist

- Create your plan to eliminate acid addictions between now and Day One of the during phase.

- Try the Swish Method!

- Follow your hydration plan.

- Rewrite your goals.

- Consume three tablespoons of omega 3 and one tablespoon of saturated fats.

DAY FIVE

Get Some Sleep!

There are a lot of things we do for our body, things we put in and things we consciously leave out. But there is another quietly cleansing, resetting, detoxification tool that we take for granted and rarely consider as a part of our armory: sleep.

Like hydration, we generally just leave sleep to chance, where sleep quality and quantity are due to circumstances. You get as much as you can and just deal with fatigue if you can't. That needs to change. You must make adequate, good rest a priority. It's an absolute necessity for optimal health.

While you're venturing through the before phase, it is a great time to assess how long and how well you're sleeping, with the aim of getting at least seven hours per night during the Cleanse itself. Done right, sleep will greatly enhance the benefits of the ARC. Done wrong, you'll be fighting an uphill battle. Your health goals will be a hundred times harder to reach if you neglect sleep or take it for granted.

As you recall, the endocrine system's organs and glands regulate hormones such as cortisol, insulin, leptin, ghrelin, testosterone, estrogen, thyroid hormones, progesterone, adrenaline—and melatonin, a.k.a. the sleep hormone. Hormones influence practically every important process in your body: fat use and storage, appetite, satiety, cognition, when to feel tired, and when to wake up. It's sort of a chicken-egg situation, where poor sleep imbalances your endocrine system and an imbalanced system interferes with the duration and quality of sleep. You can't consciously balance your endocrine system. *But*, you can certainly plan to get more rest each night. If so, you'll use more fat for energy, have better appetite control, and have less stress.

Along with hormonal regulation, sleep plays an essential role in your body's ability to detoxify and cleanse. In a University of Pittsburg study,[1] researchers discovered that people who awakened during the first sleep cycle of the night tended to have lower levels of "natural killer cells," a.k.a. the ones that hunt down germs, bacteria, and free radicals. The conclusion: Interrupted sleep means a diminished immune response. Just one disruption is enough to do it.

Other studies have found that disturbances and poor-quality sleep increased one's risk of Crohn's disease and ulcerative colitis.[2] The explanation is that digestion, absorption, and assimilation of food requires a great deal of energy. Adequate, quality sleep ensures that your digestive organs have time for rest and repair from their hard day's work. Lack of sleep also makes us more susceptible to stress, which can significantly influence digestive symptoms as well.

You might have heard that sleep flushes out brain-degenerating toxins. I'm sure you've personally experienced what your head feels like the day after a rough night. Using state-of-the-art brain imaging, researchers from New York University found that during sleep, the brain clears out twice the amount of metabolic wastes, including amyloid beta, the proteins that form the plaque associated with Alzheimer's patients.[3]

I could go on. The point is, we need quality sleep, just as we need quality nutrition. If you combine the two, you are well on your way to optimal health.

Your Sleep Plan

Find 15 *more* minutes of sleep, either at the beginning of the night or at the end of it, working up to seven hours per night *minimum*. My sleep-expert friends recommend turning off all electronics an hour before bed. The blue light from computers and phones delays the release of darkness-activated melatonin. Good sleep hygiene habits include not exercising or eating three hours before bed, no caffeine after 3 P.M. (or at all!), not doing anything in bed besides sleep and sex, keeping regular sleep hours (bad idea: sleeping super late on the weekends; that's how Sunday night insomnia happens), and, if you have trouble falling asleep, not napping during the day.

Day Five Meal Plan

Upon Waking: Turmeric and Coconut Tea
Breakfast: Alkaline Immune-Boosting Juice
Snack: The usual
Lunch: Leftover Anti-Inflammatory Soup from last night
Snack: Leftover juice from this morning
Dinner: The usual

Your first planned juice of the before phase. I hope you've already started making juices and smoothies throughout the week, but if not, today's the day! I strongly recommend you make twice as much as you'll need so you can have another serving ready to go for your midmorning or midafternoon snack. You'll also see that you'll have a second serving of last night's soup as your lunch today. I'm big on twice the goodness for half the time and effort on the ARC.

People often stress that cooking from scratch and "living healthy" takes too much time, but simply making double what you need (where it makes sense) cuts your kitchen cooking and cleaning time in half.

ALKALINE IMMUNE-BOOSTING JUICE

Makes 2 servings

Ingredients

1 cucumber
2 celery stalks
1 tomato
1 bell pepper
1 beetroot
1 handful of cilantro
8 ounces filtered (preferably alkaline) water

Instructions

Wash all the vegetables and place in a juicer. Add the water and juice!

Day Five Checklist

- Add 15 minutes to your total sleep.
- Continue weaning off acids.
- Repeat the Swish Method.
- Follow your hydration plan.
- Rewrite your goals.
- Consume three tablespoons of omega 3 and one tablespoon of saturated fats.
- Get into juicing and the philosophy of abundance.

DAY SIX

Do a Mini Assessment

You're almost up to the main event now. Everything you've done this week has given your body a massive boost and a big helping hand toward making next week as powerful *and easy* as it can possibly be. You should be incredibly proud of yourself for the effort you've made and the nourishment and goodness you've given your body already. Well done!

Today I want you to do an assessment of your progress so far. Think about what's worked for you, and any particular challenges. Were those challenges overcome, or are you worried about them for next week? How can you smooth the logistics of meal prep and planning? Transport food to work? Get in your fats and anti-inflammatories with consistency?

One of the reasons I ask you to do a prep week is to figure all this out. The week before serves as a dress rehearsal for opening night. Of course, you'll likely have some issues. But the beautiful thing is, now that you know what they are, you can work toward fixing them.

Your Assessment Plan

If you're like most people, you had a slipup at some point this week and were knocked completely off track. Awesome! Better to have done it this week than next week. The most important thing is that you do *not* beat yourself up over it. A slipup, like everything, is a huge learning opportunity, and I really want you to focus on it for a few minutes.

The plan is to have a little therapy session with yourself. Ask yourself:

- What happened before, during, and after the slipup?

- What was the trigger? (There usually is one.)

- How did I react?

- How would I have reacted in a perfect world, if I could turn back time?

- What will I do differently next time?

Just thinking through the situation and asking these questions gives you so much more self-awareness and you'll be less likely to repeat the same slip in the near future. Every small mistake and rebellion, once understood, is a huge step forward.

Day Six Meal Plan

Upon Waking: Creamy Coconut, Turmeric, and Ginger Warmer
Breakfast: Simple Alkaline Oats
Snack: The usual
Lunch: Superfood Salad
Snack: Turmeric Roasted Nuts
Dinner: The usual

You will be getting turmeric into two of your meals today already, but see if you can sneak it in a third time. Perhaps grate some into the Superfood Salad you'll be preparing to take to lunch at work today.

SUPERFOOD SALAD

Makes 2 servings

Ingredients

½ inch gingerroot, grated
1 small garlic clove, minced
1 small bunch of parsley, finely chopped
1 carrot, grated
1 small beetroot, grated

1 handful of kale, finely chopped
1 small celery stalk, sliced
½ ripe avocado, cubed
¼ cup olive oil
1 teaspoon coconut oil
¼ lemon, juiced
Sprinkle of sea salt

Instructions

Combine the ginger, garlic, parsley, carrot, beetroot, kale, and celery in a bowl and toss.

Blend the avocado, olive oil, coconut oil, lemon juice, and salt in a blender or food processor to make a creamy green dressing. Adjust the lemon and salt to taste. Pour the dressing over the salad and enjoy.

Day Six Checklist

- Brainstorm five different ways to add turmeric and ginger to your daily diet.

- Think about your successes and mess-ups this week, and figure out how to do even better next week.

- Add 15 more minutes to your sleep tonight.

- Repeat the Swish Method.

- Follow your hydration plan.

- Rewrite your goals.

- Consume three tablespoons of omega 3 and one tablespoon of saturated fats.

DAY SEVEN

Hit on All Cylinders!

Wow, you're starting your official Cleanse tomorrow! Today is the day to get in your prep-week goodness, priming your body to do amazing things next week. The more you can prep, the easier and more powerful your Cleanse will be. Have some *extra* water, *extra* greens, a big juice, loads of quality sleep, and follow these final steps.

Do NOT Have a Last Hurrah

It's so tempting to have a "last hurrah" meal, but this is an awful idea. Loading your body with acidic toxins the day before the ARC is pretty much the most counterproductive thing you can do—and really, for what? Instead, have a meal that is going to leave you feeling happy and nourished, but don't go crazy.

Revisit Your Goals

A great way to make sure you're feeling positive, motivated, disciplined, and ready to go is to remind yourself of your *whys*. Get clarity on the reasons you're doing the Cleanse, what your goals are, and what life will be like when you achieve those goals. Take some time today to relax into the right mind-set for the seven days ahead.

Shop!

With your Cleanse starting on Saturday morning, it is critical that you go shopping for your first three days of groceries on Friday evening. The very worst thing you can do is kick off your Cleanse by realizing that you have to run to the market for missing ingredients before you make your morning juice. Nothing feels quite as motivating as filling your cart with all the goodness you'll consume. Seeing just how much food it is will reassure you that you won't go hungry. If anything, you'll think, How am I possibly going to get all this in? If you live in a city and walk to the store, you will need to bring what my New York friends call an "old lady cart," or plan on taking a taxi or Uber ride home. Check the shopping list below for items that might not be at your local store (like galangal, a root). If you can't find something, don't worry about it. The (very) few obscure ingredients are good to have, but it's not a tragedy if you can't find them. Remember, we are anti-perfectionist on the Cleanse!

The shopping list is for Days One, Two, and Three of the ARC. In the next chapter, on Day Three of the Cleanse, I'll give you the shopping list for days Four through Seven. Shopping for only three (or four) days at a time ensures that your ingredients stay fresh and that you won't feel too overwhelmed. Still, it's a lot of food, so be prepared to fill up your car trunk. All those cucumbers and bags of spinach are bulky! Once you get it all home and loaded into your fridge and pantry (you'll have to make some room!), you will stand back, look at it all, and feel so inspired to get started.

Shopping List for Days One, Two, and Three

Greens, Herbs, and Other Veggies

Arugula	1 bag or 2 bunches
Avocado	5
Beet	2
Broccoli	1 large head
Cabbage, Chinese	1 head
Carrot	7
Celery	10 stalks
Chard	1 bunch
Cilantro	1 bunch
Cucumber	7
Dill	1 bunch
Garlic	1 bulb
Kale	2 big bunches
Leek	1
Lettuce	1 head
Onion, yellow	2
Pepper, green	1
Pepper, red	3
Squash, butternut	1
Spinach	5 bags or 10 bunches
Sweet potato	1
Tomato	3

Roots

Galangal	2-inch root
Ginger	1 large root
Turmeric	2 large roots (or 5 small)

Citrus	
Lemon	3
Lime	1
Seasonings	
Cayenne	1 jar
Black pepper	1 jar/grinder
Nutmeg	1 small jar
Himalayan salt	1 jar/grinder
Sea salt	1 jar/grinder
Vanilla pod (optional)	1
Oils	
Coconut oil	1 jar
Olive oil	1 small bottle
Legumes	
Lentils, dry	2 cups
Nuts and Seeds	
Almonds (raw, unsalted)	4 ounces
Cashews (raw, unsalted)	6 ounces
Chia seeds	3 ounces
Sunflower seeds	6 ounces
Liquids	
Almond milk	2 quarts
Coconut milk	2 16-ounce cans
Coconut water	1 quart
Vegetable stock	3.5 quarts

The Night Before
The night before you start, get everything ready in the kitchen. Make sure you make it as easy as possible to get rolling the minute you wake up. Lay everything out and be meticulous. The more effort you put in the night before, the more likely you are to stick with it the next morning. If you've gone to a lot of effort to get everything prepared, you won't have any reason *not* to start the next day.

Get the Logistics Out of the Way
My final recommendation for the day before you start your ARC is to get the logistics done. Print out the recipe cards (available at www.rossbridgeford.com/arc) or copy or tag the pages in the book. Read over the recipes so you know what to expect. If you need to make any substitutions, change the ingredient list to your personal taste. If there is a particular juice, soup, or smoothie you *loved* during the week before, substitute it in. You'll find the shopping lists can be a little adaptable, so if you've already done your shopping and want to change the meal plan, don't fret, you'll still have 95 percent of what you need and you can always adjust in a few days' time when you next shop.

If you can launch your ARC with everything done and dusted so that all you have to do is implement it, no thought required, you'll find it much more easy and enjoyable. A little preparation really does go a long way.

Set the Alarm
If you have any commitments the morning of your first day, you will need a few extra minutes to get ready before you leave the house. Allow yourself an extra half hour so you can get all of your juices, smoothies, and turmeric teas made in a relaxed environment. Stress is banned during the next seven days!

Day Seven Meal Plan

Totally up to you!

Just follow your instincts and let your new habits guide you to your new favorite flavors, the recipes you've loved most this week, or any that intrigue you as you look ahead to next week.

I recommend having a juice and a smoothie today to get that extra goodness in and to practice your skills one last time before the big event. But most important, rest up and get prepared, because tomorrow is going to be *amazing*.

Day Seven Checklist

- Do your shopping!
- Repeat the Swish Method!
- Follow your hydration plan.
- Revisit, refine, and rewrite your goals.
- Consume three tablespoons of omega 3 and one tablespoon of saturated fats.
- Have a juice or smoothie.
- Get to bed nice and early to relax and get ready.

As I mentioned right at the start of this chapter, these seven days of preparation before the Cleanse itself are not mission-critical. You don't have to do this if you need to start the ARC immediately. However, if you can take these simple steps during this "Before" week, you will see a huge difference. So many of my clients reach their initial goals during these seven days, even before the Cleanse has started!

These seven "Before" days are enjoyable, they're fun, and they get your momentum going and build your confidence, where you will feel such a lift in your energy and your outlook. It works like magic.

Plus, once you've completed this "Before" week, you will have so much gusto and excitement, you'll be buzzing with anticipation to jump into the ARC! So let's get into it.

CHAPTER 12

THE SEVEN DAYS OF THE ALKALINE RESET CLEANSE

The next seven days of your life are going to completely reboot, reset, heal, nourish, and kick-start your health, and balance your Five Master Systems to create a whole-body transformation. So let's jump right in!

You already know the foods you'll be eating (your fridge should be packed with green stuff already), and that you'll be drinking lots of filtered water, taking walks, bouncing, and breathing daily. But to have an even better idea of what a day looks like, hour by hour, I've created a snapshot for you.

A TYPICAL DAY ON THE ARC

Since everyone rises at their own schedule, I'll use my own wake time as an example. I am an early riser and begin the day at 6 A.M. If you wake up later, adjust your schedule accordingly.

---

6 to 6:30 A.M.
Lemon Water and Turmeric Tea or Tonic

As soon as you wake up, you'll want to start hydrating and waking up your metabolism. The very first thing I recommend you do is make yourself a large glass of warm water with a whole lemon squeezed in.

Lemon water is immune-boosting, toxin-clearing, metabolism-stimulating, alkaline, and delicious. It's a really nice way to start the day and awaken your body. While I'm drinking the lemon water, I quickly prepare the turmeric tea of the day, be it the light Turmeric and Ginger Refresher or the comforting Creamy Turmeric and Coconut faux-latte. While I'm drinking *that*, I do the prep work (getting out the ingredients and light chopping if needed) to make . . .

---

7 A.M.
Alkaline Juice

Your first "meal" of the day is the prebreakfast alkaline juice. Having a juice first delivers a big hit of nutrients to your body, without being a challenge to digest. Without fiber, the nutrients are rapidly absorbed and disseminated throughout your body, going where they need to be with a minimum of fuss.

All of my recipes for juices (and smoothies and soups) make two servings. There is an important reason for this. You will be having the second portion of this juice later in the day as a snack. Same plan for your breakfast smoothie: one serving at mealtime, another at snack time. Your dinner soup tonight will be tomorrow's lunch. The ARC was designed with ease in mind, and the last thing I want is for you to have to clean your juicer and blender more than once per day.

Over the course of the week, you'll make six different juices, all packed with flavor and nutrients galore. After you have your first serving in the early morning, store your second serving in an airtight glass or BPA-free container in the fridge. Light, heat, and air will diminish the nutrients in the juice, so get it sealed and stored in a cold, dark place ASAP.

Next, clean the juicer. The sooner you do it, the easier the job. Don't wait for veggie pulp to harden and stick to the parts. This only takes a few minutes, and you'll be glad you got it done first thing.

7:25 A.M.
Breathing Exercises

After making your tea, juicing, and cleaning, it's time to take a short break and do some deep lower-abdominal breathing. If you don't recall the exercises I described in Chapter 10, flip back to page 101 and review. If you go right from rinsing the juicer into breathing, you'll come to associate the two, and these exercises will become part of your morning routine. Don't blow them off! They take five minutes and offer powerful support to your lymphatic system, which is going to be working overtime helping remove all the stored toxins from your body.

7:30 A.M.
Breakfast Smoothie and Supplements

By now you've been awake for an hour and a half and have had a lot to drink, but you haven't had anything to "eat" yet and are probably getting hungry. Take out your blender and ingredients to make your smoothie for the day (half now, half stored for later), a big, nourishing, filling alkaline mix of yum. Of the five smoothies you'll make this week, nearly all of them have some combination of avocado, cucumber, greens, roots, nuts, seeds, nut milk, coconut oil, and coconut water—all good things. Of course, if you want to throw in your other favorite ARC-approved ingredients (no fruit, of course), you can add a handful. The sky is the limit with smoothies.

After you finish the smoothie, store your second serving in a glass or BPA-free plastic container, and clean your blender. Quick tip: If you put some water and dish soap in your blender and pulse for a few seconds, it'll be easier to clean. Put all your juicer and blender parts away so they are good to go tomorrow morning. Congrats! It's not even 8 A.M., and you've already finished two-thirds of the day's "cooking" and cleaning. How great is that?

With a nice full stomach, it's a good time to take half of your daily supplements, since vitamins and oils can be hard on an empty stomach. Ideally, you have been taking your supplements for a week already. If not, get into the swing of it now. (Go back to page 96 for an at-a-glance list of all the ones I recommend.)

8:30 A.M. to noon
Morning Hydration

After you've digested your smoothie, make a point of getting in some of your 100 ounces per day of filtered water, perhaps with green powder or herbal tea. If you can down 50 ounces before noon, you are setting yourself up for an energized afternoon and evening.

10:30 A.M.
Midmorning Juice

Once you start to notice your mental or physical energy lag, or you just feel like something delicious, have your second serving of the already prepared juice. If at all possible, take it out of the fridge to come to room temperature before drinking for better digestion. It's not a deal breaker, but if you can swing it, please do.

Noon
Lunch

For lunch, you'll make your first serving of alkaline soup. If you planned well, you made this soup for dinner last night or anytime last week and can now pull it out of the freezer to heat and eat. I often increase the ingredients in the recipe to make three servings, in case I want an additional midafternoon snack. (The soups on the ARC are never wasted; someone at home will tuck into it!)

In the early part of Cleanse week, most people do feel their energy dip in the midafternoon, so having an extra cup of warming, soothing soup more than does the trick and brings your energy back up nicely.

12:30 to 4 P.M.
Afternoon Hydration

Aim to consume another 50 ounces of filtered water (plain or green powdered), herbal tea, or turmeric tonic between lunch and dinner prep. I will keep repeating it, but you simply cannot skimp on proper hydration during the week. *It is so critical.* Cleansing without hydration is like a salad without greens. It is still tasty and pretty good, but nowhere near as powerful.

3:30 P.M.
Midafternoon Smoothie

Have the second smoothie portion now, and/or that extra cup of your lunch soup. Some people are too full from lunch and hydrating to down their afternoon smoothie. It's okay to leave it properly sealed in the fridge and have it for tomorrow's breakfast smoothie.

5 to 6 P.M.
Dinner and Supplements

For dinner you will likely have your second serving of soup. If you're feeling adventurous, energized, and creative, you might make a different soup, and keep the second serving for tomorrow's lunchtime or an emergency snack. Remember, all of these soups will keep in the fridge for 48 hours or in the freezer for up to three months.

The reason I suggest you might have a different soup at dinnertime is because it's often nice to have one of the light, raw, completely blended smooth soups at lunchtime, and then have a more traditional, chunky, warm soup at dinner, where you have something to chew (albeit pretty softly stewed vegetables).

Your brain gets a psychological boost from eating something familiar and "normal." When you have just liquids for seven days, your brain can play tricks on you and make you have some unusual cravings for solid food, and I find that having a chunky soup (even if it's blended) can immediately put these cravings to bed and satisfy your brain.

But if you're happy with your lunchtime soup, definitely feel free to stick with it for dinner. My constant refinements of the ARC over the past seven years are all about balancing optimal benefits with speed and ease. The same soup twice a day means that much less "cooking" and cleanup time. If you've been keeping track of all your kitchen time, you'll find that you've spent no more than an hour total preparing your meals. Happy days!

After dinner, with a nice full belly, is a good time to have your second round of daily supplements, especially those healthy fats which love to be digested with food rather than on an empty stomach.

8 P.M.

Breathing Exercises

I often practice the lymphatic breathing exercise when I get into bed, to put a capper on the day. Before you begin your overnight repair, this stimulation of the lymphatic system is incredibly powerful.

10 P.M.

Bedtime

Between dinner and bedtime, you should continue to hydrate gently, sipping on more lemon water, herbal teas, or mixed green powder, if you like. Don't chug down water before bed unless you fancy a midnight toilet trip. Plus, you need to start being gentle on your body now as it falls into your natural circadian rhythm and begins preparing for your overnight detox. If you can, continue the practice of rewriting your goals—for the Cleanse and big-picture ones—before bed. It's a good habit to form generally, but I find it especially useful during the Cleanse. Writing down your goals for the next day really focuses your mind and raises both your motivation and confidence. It also gives your subconscious a chance to embed your goals during your seven to eight hours of quality sleep.

So that is a "typical" day on the Cleanse. However, you should know . . .

THERE IS NO SUCH THING AS A TYPICAL DAY ON THE ARC

The schedule might be the same, but each person, on each day, will have a different experience. Some will kick off and experience amazing energy from the very first juice and never look back. Some might not get that energy hit until Day Five or Six. Some might track their journey as starting from the bottom and zooming straight up. Others may go through ups and downs throughout the week. You might have aches and pains—signs of deep detox and your body releasing long-stored acids—but your best friend might not have a single pang. You might never feel hungry, but your partner might crave juices and smoothies all day long. We are each unique and we all have a completely different body, metabolism, and health history. Someone might start the Cleanse on the back of a decade's 10-cup-a-day coffee habit. Some have been knocking back a liter of soda a day. They will have different challenges than someone who has been eating and living clean for the same length of time.

Use your experience! Pay attention to how your energy, appetite, and detox symptoms change as the week goes on. Your health will evolve right before your eyes, in a dramatically brief period of time. Everyone—and I mean every single person of the thousands I've coached through this—are thrilled by how they feel by Day Five or Six and are grateful for what they've been through and learned along the way.

Remember, the one rule to rule them all about the ARC: It's easy and fun! You are allowed to swap something you don't like for a recipe or Triple A ingredient you love. Don't feel like you have to suffer through it, gritting your teeth the whole way. Just make a different smoothie. It's okay! As long as you don't eat solid food, stick to the ingredients and recipes, and avoid the acid-forming substances, you will reap the benefits of the Cleanse. If you feel hungry, have another juice, another cup of soup, another tea. If you feel tired, take a catnap. If you feel stiff, do some yoga or get a massage. Massages are a wonderful way to mobilize lymph! If you can splurge, I recommend getting one on Day Three or Four.

Another add-on, along with a massage, is **dry brushing**. I heartily recommend that everyone consider using a skin brush (less than $20, available at drug stores, online, anywhere, really), and use it in the morning before your shower every day. I've talked about other detoxification organs—the liver, kidneys, guts, and lungs. Your skin is also a detox organ that shouldn't be forgotten. The body eliminates toxins through your breath, urine, feces, *and sweat*. Dry brushing clears away dead cells, unblocking pores and supporting your skin to exhale and sweat more effectively. Just brush in long, fluid movements, always toward the heart, starting at your feet and moving upward.

Also, **don't skip exercise**! I didn't include exercise in the "typical day" snapshot because we're all different, with different schedules and routines. Whenever you can, take a brisk walk, do some bouncing, go for a swim, do yoga. Just spend some time every day moving your body and supporting your lymph and detoxification process. Try to plan 30 minutes to an hour of exercise into your routine—rebounding before breakfast, biking to work, walking at lunchtime, a predinner yoga class—to make sure it happens.

DETOX SYMPTOMS AND HOW TO AVOID THEM

If you've ever done any kind of cleanse or detox or have simply tried to give up caffeine or sugar before, you're likely aware of the dreaded detox symptoms.

Most common among them are headaches, nausea, flu-like symptoms, fatigue, light-headedness, acne, aches, and pains. These are all signs of your body rapidly eliminating toxins while adjusting to the withdrawal of sugar, grains, caffeine, etc.

The degree to which you might experience these symptoms is entirely personal and random. Some get all of them, while others get none. On the ARC, your chance of experiencing them is significantly diminished, since you will be flooding the body with the best weapons against withdrawal symptoms, namely antioxidants, anti-inflammatories, and alkaline-forming foods. Plus, since you are giving your body all the good stuff, your symptoms will disappear much faster than they would if you ate your normal diet and went cold turkey on coffee.

The ARC's rule "Never go hungry!" helps. One of the main reasons people have these detox symptoms, particularly fatigue, headaches, and flu-ish aches, is because they are not eating enough. On the ARC, eat as much as you like. In fact, having more of the good stuff is the antidote to feeling tired or headachy.

So before you take a pain pill, try these cures for detox symptoms:

Consume. More juice, more smoothie, more soup. My recipes are generous; you'll have plenty to enjoy at mealtime or anytime. You will always have some juice, soup, or smoothie on hand, so drink them!

Drink. Super-hydrate. The symptoms are merely a sign of your body expelling the toxins (or trying to). By consuming more food and lots more water, you help your body speed up this process.

Rest. It's not always possible if you're at work, I know. This is one of the reasons I ask people to start the Cleanse on the weekend or when you have a couple of free nonwork days to chill. Most detox symptoms come up in the first 24 to 72 hours. If you can, lie down for a nap, or go to be bed another 15 minutes earlier to give the body even more overnight detox time.

Eat. If you're really desperate and feel like actual food might help, cut an avocado in half and top it with chopped tomato, olive oil, salt, and pepper. It's not liquid, but it's not exactly solid either, and it might give you a psychological lift to make you forget those pesky detox symptoms.

Remember, most people get very mild symptoms, if any. And no one in all my years of teaching the Cleanse has suffered so intensely that they had to stop. In fact, they were even more committed to the Cleanse, because their symptoms were signs that it was working. If you don't experience symptoms, don't worry that the Cleanse isn't working. It is! You'll experience other clues of the benefits in greater energy, clarity, or a feeling of lightness and brightness.

Without further ado, here's **your Alkaline Reset Cleanse**, broken down **day by day**, with recipes, your final shopping list, and some insight into what you'll likely experience as you go along.

The Alkaline Reset Cleanse Meal Plan

	Saturday	Sunday	Monday	Tuesday	Wednesday	Thursday	Friday
Upon Waking	Turmeric & Ginger Refresher Tea	Creamy Turmeric & Coconut Tea	Turmeric & Ginger Refresher Tea	Creamy Turmeric & Coconut Tea	Turmeric & Ginger Refresher Tea	Creamy Turmeric & Coconut Tea	Turmeric & Ginger Refresher Tea
Prebreakfast	Live Energized Green Juice	Alkaline High-Energy Juice	Anti-Inflammation Juice	Blood-Builder Juice	Digestion Juice	Live Energized Green Juice	Immune-Boosting Juice
Breakfast	Core Green Alkaline Smoothie	Alkaline Avocado Power Smoothie	All-Day Energy Smoothie	Antioxidant Green Smoothie	Alkaline Avocado Power Smoothie	Anti-Inflammatory Smoothie	Antioxidant Green Smoothie
Snack	Live Energized Green Juice	Alkaline High-Energy Juice	Anti-Inflammation Juice	Blood-Builder Juice	Digestion Juice	Live Energized Green Juice	Immune-Boosting Juice
Lunch	Warming Alkaline Broccoli Soup	Carrot & Ginger Soup	Soothing Gut-Healing Soup	Warming Squash Soup	Immune-Boosting Soup	Anti-Inflammatory Soup	Cucumber & Watercress Soup
Snack	Core Green Alkaline Smoothie	Alkaline Avocado Power Smoothie	All-Day Energy Smoothie	Antioxidant Green Smoothie	Alkaline Avocado Power Smoothie	Anti-Inflammatory Smoothie	Antioxidant Green Smoothie
Dinner	Carrot & Ginger Soup	Soothing Gut-Healing Soup	Warming Squash Soup	Immune-Boosting Soup	Anti-Inflammatory Soup	Cucumber & Watercress Soup	Alkaline Raw Soup

Daily Drinks: Between 2 and 4 liters of filtered water daily

DAY ONE
Saturday (or Your "Saturday")

You've arrived! Today is the day you kick off, and it's so important that you start the day right, positively and proactively. If you've done your shopping and preparations the night before, getting started should be a breeze.

Today I want you to focus on following the steps and paying attention to the little details. Think about how the Cleanse is working in your life. Is the juicing easy? Is it too noisy too early in the morning? Does it wake up your kids? Do you need to adjust for that? How long is it between "meals" before you begin to feel hungry? Do you need to make more each time for extra snacks? Be inquisitive and aware throughout the day so you can spot ways to optimize and personalize the Cleanse to suit you and your life.

I recommend that you write down your exercise and breathing schedule, and stick to the plan as closely as possible. This will give you a ton of confidence going into tomorrow.

One housekeeping note: Today only, you will make two soups. (If you happen to have leftover soup from prep week, you can substitute that for one of the two recipes below, or just make both of these.) Choose to save the second portion of one soup for lunch tomorrow and put the second portion of the other in the freezer to heat and eat as needed anytime.

Day One Meal Plan

Upon waking: Lemon water
Prebreakfast tea: Turmeric and Ginger Refresher Tea
Prebreakfast juice: Live Energized Green Juice
Breakfast smoothie: Core Green Alkaline Smoothie
Midmorning juice: Live Energized Green Juice
Lunch: Warming Alkaline Broccoli Soup
Midafternoon smoothie: Core Green Alkaline Smoothie
Dinner: Carrot and Ginger Soup

TURMERIC AND GINGER REFRESHER TEA

Makes 2 servings

Ingredients

1 inch fresh turmeric root, peeled and grated
1 inch fresh gingerroot, peeled and grated
2 cups filtered (or, preferably, alkaline) water
1 lemon

Instructions

Put the turmeric and ginger into a pot with the water.

Bring to a simmer for a few minutes until the water turns orange.

Pour into a mug and squeeze in the lemon. Watch with fascination as the orange water turns bright yellow.

Drink warm.

LIVE ENERGIZED GREEN JUICE

Makes 2 servings

Ingredients

1 cucumber
2 celery stalks
2 handfuls of spinach
2 handfuls of kale
2 handfuls of lettuce
1 carrot
½ lemon for squeezing
Filtered water to add hydration (optional)

Instructions

Juice all the ingredients, and then squeeze in a little lemon before serving.

CORE GREEN ALKALINE SMOOTHIE

Makes 2 servings

Ingredients

½ avocado
1 cucumber
½ cup filtered water or more to taste
2 handfuls of spinach
2 handfuls of lettuce

½ bell pepper
1 tomato
½ inch gingerroot
1 cm turmeric
Squeeze of fresh lemon

Instructions

Start by blending the avocado, cucumber, and water to form a liquid base, which makes it easier to blend everything else.

Next, add the spinach, lettuce, bell pepper, tomato, ginger, and turmeric in that order. If you don't have a high-powered blender, you might need to grate the ginger and turmeric first.

Squeeze in a little lemon for zing, and serve.

WARMING ALKALINE BROCCOLI SOUP

Makes 2 servings

Ingredients

1 large head of broccoli, florets only
½ avocado
½ cup organic low-sodium vegetable stock
1 cucumber

1 handful of spinach
1 handful of arugula
1 garlic clove
½ inch fresh gingerroot, sliced very thin
Squeeze of lemon or lime juice

Instructions

Steam the broccoli until it's bright green (7 or 8 minutes on the stove top; 3 minutes in the microwave).

Blend the avocado and vegetable stock.

Add the cucumber, spinach, arugula, garlic, and ginger to the blender and blend. Then add the warmed broccoli and blend.

The broccoli should warm the soup, but if you need it warmer, put the mixture into a saucepan for a few minutes.

Serve with a squeeze of lemon or lime on top.

CARROT AND GINGER SOUP

Makes 2 servings

Ingredients

1 tablespoon coconut oil
1 small yellow onion, chopped
2 garlic cloves, chopped
1 leek, washed and finely sliced
1 celery stalk, finely chopped
4 cups roughly chopped carrots

1 tablespoon fresh grated ginger
1 teaspoon fresh grated turmeric or
½ teaspoon dry
6 cups (48 ounces) organic, low-sodium vegetable stock
½ cup chopped cilantro
Sea salt and black pepper to taste

Instructions

Gently warm the coconut oil in a saucepan. Add the onion, garlic, leek, and celery. Cook for 3 to 4 minutes.

Add the carrots, ginger, and turmeric and stir for 1 to 2 minutes before adding the stock.

Bring to a boil, then reduce the heat to a simmer for 10 to 12 minutes until the carrots are tender.

Remove the mixture from the heat and stir in the cilantro. Either transfer to a blender and blend the soup until smooth, or use an immersion blender to blend in the pot. Add salt and pepper to taste. Serve warm.

DAY TWO
Sunday (or Your "Sunday")

Today you should wake up feeling refreshed and alert. If detox symptoms are kicking in, megahydrate and megafuel. Feel free to just jump right into any leftover soups, juices, or smoothies from yesterday. Revisiting your goals is so important whether you're dealing with detox symptoms or not. Keep going, but go easy on yourself with lots of rest, some extra sleep, more food, and more hydration. Be kind to yourself.

For most people, if you started the Cleanse on a Saturday, tomorrow will mean going back to work, but *not* returning to your usual workday eating habits. If you have a plan to handle the change, you will be fine. Tonight, do some basic prep.

The three challenges of working while cleansing: (1) mornings will be rushed; (2) you won't have access to your kitchen and equipment all day; and (3) you'll need to transport your snacks and lunch with you to your workplace. The last one is easy: Investing in some good airtight containers and a portable cooler bag (an "esky" as we say in Australian) is a smart idea. As for the other two . . .

In the morning, you have a lot to do before you get out the door, namely, making your tea, juices, and smoothies for the day and packing up your lunch soup. Any prep you can do tonight for tomorrow will streamline the process. Prewash and chop your veggies so that in the morning, you can just throw them all into the juicer and blender. Some people like to make the next day's juices and smoothies and refrigerate overnight, which is also fine. Others do a combination of both. Whatever you choose, just do something in advance to make it easier on yourself. There is nothing worse than being at work, out of the house, and hungry with no access to a Cleanse meal. Believe me, it'll be hard to find a Cleanse-friendly meal in restaurants, shops, and cafés. Even juice and smoothie stores might sneak in fruit or syrups or not use organic ingredients (preferred, but not crucial if you wash your veggies well).

Even if you do prepare, tomorrow morning might seem hectic. I promise, you will get better at this, and by the end of the week, it'll become a natural routine.

Day Two Meal Plan

Upon waking: Lemon water
Prebreakfast tea: Creamy Turmeric and Coconut Tea
Prebreakfast juice: Alkaline High-Energy Juice
Breakfast smoothie: Alkaline Avocado Power Smoothie
Midmorning juice: Alkaline High-Energy Juice
Lunch: Carrot and Ginger Soup (leftover from yesterday)
Midafternoon smoothie: Alkaline Avocado Power Smoothie
Dinner: Soothing Gut-Healing Soup

CREAMY TURMERIC AND COCONUT TEA

Makes 2 servings

Ingredients

1 ½ inches fresh gingerroot
1 inch fresh turmeric root
2 teaspoons coconut oil
1 cup full-fat coconut milk

1 cup coconut or filtered water
1 teaspoon cloves
1 vanilla pod (optional)

Instructions

Peel the ginger and turmeric and grate into a mortar.

Add the coconut oil and, using the pestle, turn it into a beautiful orange-yellow paste.

Pour the coconut cream and water into a saucepan. Spoon in the paste and add the cloves and vanilla pod.

Simmer for 4 to 5 minutes.

Serve warm, straining if you wish.

ALKALINE HIGH-ENERGY JUICE

Makes 2 servings

Ingredients

1 cucumber
2 celery stalks, chopped
2 large leaves of Chinese cabbage
3 large leaves of chard

2 small beets with greens
2 large handfuls of baby spinach
1 inch gingerroot
1 cup coconut water or filtered water

Instructions

Juice all the ingredients, add water to taste and enjoy!

ALKALINE AVOCADO POWER SMOOTHIE

Makes 2 servings

Ingredients

1 avocado, roughly chopped
½ teaspoon vegetable stock
1 cucumber, roughly chopped
2 tomatoes, roughly chopped
½ red pepper, roughly chopped

1 handful of spinach
1 lime
1 tablespoon Udo's Choice oil or flax oil (optional)

Instructions

Place the avocado and stock in a blender and process into a paste.

Add the cucumber, tomatoes, and pepper and blend into a liquid.

Add the spinach and lime.

Blend in the oil, if using, and serve in a tall glass.

SOOTHING GUT-HEALING SOUP

Makes 2 servings

Ingredients

1 cup dry lentils (or one 12-ounce can, drained and rinsed)
4 garlic cloves, chopped
1 yellow onion, chopped
1 tablespoon coconut oil
1 large sweet potato, peeled and chopped
2 carrots, peeled and chopped
1 cup organic low-sodium vegetable stock

1 avocado
1 red bell pepper, chopped
1 large handful of spinach
2 tablespoons dill, chopped, plus sprigs for garnish
1 handful of cashews, roughly chopped
Salt and pepper to taste
1 teaspoon olive oil

Instructions

Prepare the lentils according to the package instructions and set aside. (This step takes 20 to 30 minutes, the longest step in the recipe.)

Gently warm the garlic and onion in coconut oil in a large pot for 3 minutes until browned.

Add the sweet potato and carrots. Stir until evenly coated and the flavors come together, about 2 to 4 minutes.

Add the stock and simmer for 10 minutes until the vegetables are warmed through but not overcooked to retain as many nutrients as possible.

Add the lentils. Cook for another 5 minutes.

Either transfer the mixture to a blender in batches or use an immersion blender to blend the contents in the pot. Add the avocado, pepper, spinach, and dill and blend.

Garnish with a few springs of dill and cashews. Serve warm with a drizzle of olive oil on top.

DAY THREE

Monday (or Your First Day of the Workweek)

Your first workday on the Cleanse! If you prepared your meals or ingredients last night, or got up a few minutes early this morning, you will be fine. And if you didn't, you will learn to do so moving forward. In no time, you'll be a pro, and you'll have your daytime meals packed in your cooler bag and ready to go like it's second nature. This is very important! The biggest risk of cleansing on a workday schedule is that you'll get hungry and have nothing available to "eat." If you think it wise, pack *extra* smoothies and soup portions to prevent that from happening.

By Day Three, detox symptoms (if you had any; remember, 65 percent of people don't) will be pretty much over. You should be feeling vibrant, energized, and focused, and motivated to keep the goodness going!

Day Three Meal Plan

Upon waking: Lemon water
Prebreakfast tea: Turmeric and Ginger Refresher Tea (page 155)
Prebreakfast juice: Anti-Inflammation Juice
Breakfast smoothie: All-Day Energy Smoothie
Midmorning juice: Anti-Inflammation Juice
Lunch: Soothing Gut-Healing Soup (leftover from yesterday)

Midafternoon smoothie: All-Day Energy Smoothie
Dinner: Warming Squash Soup

ANTI-INFLAMMATION JUICE

Makes 2 servings

Ingredients

1 inch fresh turmeric
1 inch fresh ginger
½ inch fresh galangal (only if you can find it; otherwise, no worries!)

1 handful of spinach
1 handful of kale
1 cucumber
1 cup filtered (preferably alkaline) water

Instructions

Wash all the ingredients and juice them in the order listed. Mix in the water and enjoy!

ALL-DAY ENERGY SMOOTHIE

Makes 2 servings

Ingredients

½ cup soaked almonds
¼ cup soaked cashews
½ ripe avocado
1 cup almond milk
½ cucumber

3 tablespoons coconut oil
2 handfuls of spinach
1 handful of kale
1 tablespoon sunflower seeds
1 tablespoon chia seeds

Instructions

If you are reading this in advance, soak the almonds and cashews for an hour or, preferably, overnight. If you want to make the recipe now, soak them for at least 20 minutes!

Blend the avocado, almond milk, and cucumber.

Add the coconut oil, spinach, and kale.

Add the soaked nuts and sunflower and chia seeds, and blend until smooth. Enjoy!

WARMING SQUASH SOUP

Makes 2 servings

Ingredients

1 ¼ cups organic low-sodium vegetable stock
1 large butternut squash, deseeded and chopped into small chunks (keep the seeds for roasting, if you like; they're delicious!)
1 yellow onion, sliced
1 12-ounce can coconut milk
Himalayan salt and cracked black pepper to taste
Sprinkle of nutmeg

Instructions

Place the stock in a pot and bring to a boil.

Add the squash, onion, coconut milk, salt, and pepper. Once boiling, reduce the mixture to a simmer. Simmer until the squash is soft, about 10 minutes. Transfer to a blender in batches, or use an immersion blender. Blend until smooth.

Serve warm with a sprinkle of nutmeg and a smile!

Based on how things went today, you will know what preparation adjustments you'll want to make for tomorrow, how hungry you get (and, therefore, how much food you need to bring to work with you tomorrow), and how much time you need in the morning to get everything ready before work.

Your fridge has been cleared out already! It might seem like a miracle that you actually consumed all that food. But you did. Every single nutrient in every leaf of spinach has been put to good use inside you.

Today you will need to restock your fridge with even more powerful foods to keep your Cleanse and transformation going for Days Four through Seven. Shopping only twice in the week is probably less than you were doing before. You're definitely spending less time and money in restaurants and bodegas. As with all the recipes and meal plans, the following shopping list can be downloaded at www.rossbridgeford.com/arc. Again, bring a cart or car or friend with you to the store. You might be bursting with energy now, but this is still a lot to carry home by yourself!

SHOPPING LIST FOR DAYS FOUR THROUGH SEVEN

Since you will have leftover nuts, seeds, seasonings, and oils, you won't need to buy those ingredients again. Notice how your pantry is already changing after the previous week and this week? Out with acid-forming foods, and in with healthy oils, containers of seeds and nuts, beans and lentils, liters of coconut water, and cans of beans and coconut milk. I get inspired to create new menus just by looking in the pantry.

Greens, Herbs, and Other Veggies	
Avocado	4
Beet	1
Broccoli	8 heads
Cabbage, white	1 head
Carrots	7
Celery	8 stalks
Cilantro	1 large bunch
Cucumber	10
Garlic	1 bulb
Kale	2 bunches
Kale, Tuscan	1 bunch
Lettuce	1 head
Mint	1 bunch
Onion, red	2
Onion, yellow	1
Parsley, flat-leaf	1 bunch
Pepper, red	3
Potato, red bliss	1
Pumpkin	2 12-ounce cans (or 1 small)
Squash, butternut	1
Scallion	2 bunches
Spinach	5 bags or 10 bunches
Tomato	10
Watercress	3 bunches

Roots	
Ginger	1 large root
Turmeric	3 large roots (or 7 small)
Citrus	
Lemon	4
Lime	1
Seasonings	
Cumin	1 jar
Mustard seeds	1 jar
Legumes	
Cannellini beans (canned)	4 cups
Lentils, dry	1 cup
Liquids	
Coconut cream	1 12-ounce can
Coconut milk	2 12-ounce cans
Coconut water	2 liters
Vegetable stock	3 liters
Misc	
Bragg Liquid Aminos	1 6-ounce bottle

DAY FOUR

Congrats! You are halfway there, and all the heavy lifting (shopping, detox symptoms, getting used to the logistics) is behind you! Your energy should be rising and sustaining by now, and you're probably experiencing much greater mental clarity and none of the afternoon energy dips. The results from here will just continue to grow and grow.

By now you understand how the recipes are created. The juices usually have a combination of high-water veggies, plus roots, plus leaves. The smoothies include avocado, plus high-water veggies, leaves, and protein—and fats-packed seeds and nuts. The soups are like grandma used to make, just throwing a lot of the good stuff into a pot to warm and comfort you in more ways than one. After four days of intense infusion of nutrients, your taste has already started to change, making you more sensitive to subtle flavors in these recipes and turned off by the blown-out, oversalted, high sugar content in acid-forming foods. Your appetite is also changing. The cravings for calorie-rich snacks in the afternoon have disappeared, just like the habit for munching on chips and popcorn after dinner. Once you put down your spoons after dinner, you are content and happy not to "eat" again until your morning tea. The reason for the absence of cravings? Your hormones are balancing and your gut is absorbing more nutrients than ever, so your body doesn't need to send the signal, "Feed me!" to the brain. You are getting more of everything you need, and nothing you don't need.

Day Four Meal Plan

Upon waking: Lemon water
Prebreakfast tea: Creamy Turmeric and Coconut Tea (page 159)
Prebreakfast juice: Blood-Builder Juice
Breakfast smoothie: Antioxidant Green Smoothie (page 119)
Midmorning juice: Blood-Builder Juice
Lunch: Warming Squash Soup (leftover from yesterday)
Midafternoon smoothie: Antioxidant Green Smoothie
Dinner: Immune-Boosting Soup

BLOOD-BUILDER JUICE

Makes 2 servings

Ingredients

1 cucumber
2 large handfuls of spinach
1 handful of parsley
1 celery stalk

Instructions

Juice! Drink! Enjoy!

IMMUNE-BOOSTING SOUP

Makes 2 servings

Ingredients

1 tablespoon coconut oil
1 red onion, diced
4 garlic cloves, minced
2 tablespoons ginger, finely grated
2 medium carrots, diced
4 cups cooked or canned cannellini
beans, drained and rinsed
1 teaspoon turmeric powder

32 ounces organic low-sodium
vegetable stock
1 small bunch Tuscan kale, roughly
chopped
1 handful of flat-leaf parsley, roughly
chopped
Splash of olive oil
Salt and pepper to taste

Instructions

Warm the coconut oil in a large pan, then add the onion. Cook until translucent and slightly browned. Add the garlic and ginger and cook for 2 to 3 minutes.

Add the carrots, beans, and turmeric. Cook for 3 or 4 minutes before adding the stock.

Bring the mixture to a boil, then reduce to a simmer for 10 minutes.

Add the kale and parsley, stirring through and cooking until the kale is slightly soft.

Ladle the soup into bowls and top with a drizzle of olive oil and season with salt and pepper to taste. (That's right—no blending tonight!)

DAY FIVE

You're getting toward the end of the week and you can probably feel your body returning to how it *should* be. Most people have no idea how great their bodies are meant to feel, but you are getting the idea. For most, Day Five is when the biggest benefits start to emerge. Days One through Four are good, but Days Five through Seven lift things up to another level. Now more than ever, remember to keep up your hydration, don't skip the breathing exercises, keep moving every day for at least 30 minutes, take your supplements, rewrite your goals, and get some sleep!

Day Five Meal Plan

Upon waking: Lemon water
Prebreakfast tea: Turmeric and Ginger Refresher Tea (page 155)
Prebreakfast juice: Digestion Juice
Breakfast smoothie: Alkaline Avocado Power Smoothie (page 160)
Midmorning juice: Digestion Juice
Lunch: Immune-Boosting Soup (leftover from yesterday)
Midafternoon smoothie: Alkaline Avocado Power Smoothie (page 160)
Dinner: Anti-Inflammatory Soup (page 132)

DIGESTION JUICE

Makes 2 servings

Ingredients

1/3 head of white cabbage, leaves separated and cleaned
1 handful of spinach
½ cucumber
½ inch ginger
½ lemon
1 small bunch fresh mint

Instructions

You tell me. I'm sure you know what to do by now. Wash and juice!

DAY SIX

You're on the home stretch now and are well into the swing of it. You can consider yourself an expert at juicing and blending. You probably have the process of making the recipes (from chopping to cleaning) down to a fine art.

These final two days of the ARC are a beautiful combination of a sense of achievement and accomplishment, how amazing your body feels, how you look in the mirror, and a host of positive, heightened emotions. You feel like you can do anything, and you probably can (within reason!).

Day Six Meal Plan

Upon waking: Lemon water
Prebreakfast tea: Creamy Turmeric and Coconut Tea (page 159)
Prebreakfast juice: Live Energized Juice (page 155)
Breakfast smoothie: Anti-Inflammatory Smoothie
Midmorning juice: Live Energized Juice (page 155)
Lunch: Anti-Inflammatory Soup (leftover from yesterday)
Midafternoon smoothie: Anti-Inflammatory Smoothie
Dinner: Cucumber and Watercress Soup

ANTI-INFLAMMATORY SMOOTHIE

Makes 2 servings

Ingredients

1 inch fresh ginger, grated
1 inch fresh turmeric, grated
1 small avocado
1 cup coconut water
1 handful of baby spinach
1 handful of watercress or arugula

½ red pepper
1 big handful of flat-leaf parsley or cilantro
1 big pinch of cayenne
Salt

Instructions

Blend the ginger and turmeric in the blender. Add the avocado and coconut water. Blend.

Add the remaining ingredients and blend until smooth(ie).

CUCUMBER AND WATERCRESS SOUP

Makes 2 servings

Ingredients

½ bunch scallions, chopped
1 large cucumber, deseeded and chopped
2 bunches watercress
4 cups (32 ounces) organic low-sodium vegetable stock
Himalayan salt and fresh ground pepper to taste

Instructions

Place all the ingredients in a blender and process until smooth.

Serve chilled with an ice cube in the middle of the bowl.

DAY SEVEN

The last day! Just enjoy it and be sure to make a plan for how you're going to reward yourself tomorrow. Another benefit to starting on a Saturday is that your first day after finishing is also on the weekend, so you can go and have lots of fun to celebrate finishing. Be sure to read the next chapter about the Rest of Your Alkaline Life before you make reservations.

Today I'm giving you recipes you've made before (with one exception). Revisiting them will feel like a reunion with old friends. The only new recipe is your dinner soup, perhaps the easiest one to make, and a favorite of mine. Finish strong, and you will feel even more proud of yourself and what you've accomplished!

Day Seven Meal Plan

Upon waking: Lemon water
Prebreakfast tea: Turmeric and Ginger Refresher Tea (page 155)
Prebreakfast juice: Alkaline Immune-Boosting Juice (page 136)
Breakfast smoothie: Antioxidant Green Smoothie (page 119)
Midmorning juice: Alkaline Immune-Boosting Juice
Lunch: Cucumber and Watercress Soup (leftover from yesterday)
Midafternoon smoothie: Antioxidant Green Smoothie
Dinner: Alkaline Raw Soup

ALKALINE RAW SOUP

Makes 2 servings

Ingredients

1 avocado
½ cup organic low-sodium vegetable stock
2 scallions
½ red or green pepper
1 cucumber

2 handfuls of spinach
½ clove garlic
Juice of 1 lemon or lime
A few springs of cilantro and/or parsley (optional)
A dash of cumin (optional)

Instructions

Blend the avocado and stock to form a paste, then throw everything else in the blender. Blend until soup! Add cilantro, parsley, and cumin for garnish.

Wow! How Easy Was That?

With everything I teach, I make my lessons and recipes as easy as possible while netting you the biggest benefits. Personally, I consider this Cleanse to be one of my greatest achievements. And I hope you will consider the experience of doing the Cleanse and taking on challenges day by day to become one of yours. Now that you've been through it and have witnessed the benefits in your own body, you can see how rebalancing your Five Master Systems by following the Triple A Method framework really is the key to maximizing your health. By having alkaline, anti-inflammatory, and antioxidant juices, smoothies, and soups, you really can reset your body on a cellular level and live energized with all the vitality and clarity you deserve.

You can also attest that a cleanse doesn't have to be about suffering to be effective. You can get incredible results with a plan that is easy and fun. As amazing as you feel now—proud, light, positive, energized, strong, confident, vital, and strong—you have no idea what's coming in the weeks ahead. Day Seven is the last day of the Cleanse, but the transformation of your health and outlook is only just beginning.

One of the most satisfying parts of coaching so many people through the Alkaline Reset Cleanse is that they stay active in the "Cleanse Community" on my website, where I've heard about their dramatic results *after* their ARC experience.

In almost every case, the results multiply and amplify for weeks and months after they've finished. It takes seven days to reboot. And then, when all Five Master Systems are back up and running in balance, the weight will seem to fall off on its own. Your skin will clear. Your sleep will be easy and deep. Chronic ailments will improve. Your body wants to be healthy. Now it can be.

Of course, you can't finish the Cleanse, go back to the standard modern diet, and expect to see those results. You'll just unbalance yourself all over again. Some clients continue eating green while reintroducing meat at dinner and a cup of coffee in the morning. Others like their glass of wine or three a week. I want you to know that it's okay to enjoy wine, coffee, meat, and even sugar and dairy on occasion, if you are sticking with Triple A foods and drinks the majority of the time. I think I've made the point that shooting for perfection is the fastest way to fail. The post-Cleanse protocol is covered in the next chapter, so turn the page (in life and in the book) and read on!

Juanita's Story

I started the ARC with Ross because I was diagnosed with lupus. The doctor told me there was no cure, that it would be an ongoing disorder that would affect the rest of my life. Steroids every day, pain every day, going into the hospital for three to five days because the pain would be unbearable. That would be my existence.

At one point, I was having to take so many steroids, it felt like my body just shut down. I couldn't walk properly. My head was dizzy, I couldn't focus. I couldn't do my job. I was all over the place. I did not want to accept that this was it. If I did, it would have felt like my life was done. I felt like I might as well die if the future was nothing but meds and suffering.

I was sure there would be an answer with food and nutrition. After a very bad day, I said, "That's it." I went straight to Ross and started the Cleanse "before" week. And before I knew it, everything just went away.

I was pain free! Just that speaks for itself! The flare-ups were no longer happening and all of my inflammation has gone, too.

So the Cleanse *works*! After completing it, I realized how much weight was just dropping off me. I weighed myself after 30 days and I had lost more than 20 pounds! People think I'm younger than I am now, too, so it's just awesome!

My future is now looking very bright. From being in pain every day and on horrendous amounts of steroids to being pain free, medication free, lighter, more energized, and feeling great.

And this year, I am going to be fulfilling one of my ambitions that I never thought possible a year ago: I will be hiking Mount Fuji!

CHAPTER 13

THE REST OF YOUR ALKALINE LIFE

Congrats! You have wiped the slate clean, giving yourself a fresh start. You have reset your Five Master Systems and cleansed your digestive system. You feel phenomenal, and now you understand what your body needs and that you hold the key to a lifetime of abundance, freedom, and vitality.

Welcome to Day Zero—in other words, the opportunity of a lifetime.

Day Zero is the morning after Day Seven of the ARC. This morning bliss marks the end of your seven days of liquids and the beginning of the after phase and your new life. Your pH system is no longer using up all your energy to buffer strong acid foods and their toxic, acidic by-products or your alkaline mineral reserves. It can now redirect those minerals to where they can do good. As a result, you have excess energy reserves, ready to sustain you beautifully throughout the day.

Revel in your excess energy, strength, and connection to your mind, body, and spirit. You are now primed and ready to experience more impactful benefits, with no extra effort. And you did all that in just seven days!

Sam's Story

As a dancer, my weight has always been an issue. My first diet was at 11 years old. Losing weight, making sure you had your body a certain way and were able to perform meant you basically couldn't eat anything. When you're young, you don't realize what you're doing to yourself. I described myself as a real "punisher" to my body.

And after 30 years, my body was worn out. Decades of extreme dieting left me with chronic fatigue and terrible inflammation—and in the end, I was overweight. My exhaustion was hard on my family. The lack of enthusiasm, the moodiness, not wanting to do stuff, not wanting to go out and socialize, and not being able to go on a walk.

I had to change. We have a special-needs son, so I had to do it for him.

I loaded fully into the Alkaline Reset Cleanse. With the support group and Ross backing me up, my life changed completely, and I know it will never be the same.

After days, the inflammation and pain in my foot was gone. I could go running again, and this just created more energy and more enthusiasm. The weight started to go, and the shape of my face shifted.

And the cravings! Oh my! I used to have cravings that were impossible to ignore. But these don't come along now. I feel like I've got so much more free will and now my body is telling me what it needs! People think that, to be healthy, they'll be stuck in the kitchen all day, but it's not true. Simple and easy is the way to go. Cooking every day has been a life-changer for me, too.

My family is relieved. They feel like they got their Sam back. Suddenly the shiny, sparkly person they used to know before things went south has returned.

Eugenia's Story

I have two children under seven *and* I run a small business *and* I'm general counsel attorney at an advertising agency. My schedule is at the max. I would work a long day and then I would say, "Okay, I've earned a burger and fries with milkshake."

It would really make me feel good to eat all that, even if I felt disgusting after. I would tell myself that I really needed something better, but I just couldn't get out of my own way.

Obviously, I was gaining weight. More than anything, I was exhausted. I was always tired and stressed out, which made me grumpy. I was stuck in a very negative mental space.

It was a pattern that I had to break but I didn't know how. I heard about Ross from a friend, and looked him up. I decided that I'd try the Cleanse.

In just the first seven days, I lost nine pounds. Then, in the next seven days, another 10 pounds were gone. I am a black woman and I am very curvy. It has always been hard for me to lose weight, but I did, really easily. Even better, the Cleanse changed the way I look at food, the way I respond to stress, the way I eat, and the way I prepare for my day.

The benefits keep coming weeks after the Cleanse: energy increase, weight loss, better sleep (and I mean really good sleep, the sleep that I used to have when I was young), and an improved response to stresses.

I am more energized and I feel more positive and more excited about the possibilities of what I can do. I feel proud of the diet, the nutrition that I eat. And I feel proud of myself, for *me*.

HOW TO GET THE MOST OUT OF THE CLEANSE MOVING FORWARD

As you move from the relatively strict "during" phase into, effectively, the rest of your life, the last thing you need is to feel like you're "on a diet." What you put into place now by going alkaline and being mindful of acidity, inflammation, and oxidative stress is a lifestyle, not a diet. A diet is, by nature, short term, but a lifestyle is forever. And if it's going to be forever, you might as well make it fun, easy, and achievable—and, of course, delicious.

THE TWO PRINCIPLES FOR CONTINUED SUCCESS

There are two principles that form the bedrock of my coaching:

1. The Pareto Principle, a.k.a. the 80/20 Rule

2. The Power of Simple Daily Habits

The Pareto Principle can be applied to the worlds of business, sports, science, and medicine, or, in this case, health and wellness. It was created by an engineer and marketing consultant named Joseph Juran, who called it "the laws of the vital few and the trivial many." Generally, it states that 80 percent of your rewards come from 20 percent of your efforts.

Think about that: 80 percent of the health you experience will come from 20 percent of the actions you take. So what are the "vital few" actions from the Cleanse that you will continue to take as you go forward?

My own spin on the Pareto Principle is based on my almost 15 years of coaching the alkaline lifestyle as a way of achieving and maintaining abundant health. I've found that once people hit 80 percent of their goal, the final 20 percent happens effortlessly. Foods that were so hard to say no to before suddenly become easy to reject when you're 80 percent of the way there. Once you're at 80 percent of your potential energy and vitality, you will have the momentum, the confidence, and an abundance of desire to keep on going. Good choices will become effortless.

If you finish the Cleanse and realize that you love turmeric tea instead of coffee, smoothies for breakfast, and 100 ounces of water per day, just continue those efforts and expect to get 80 percent of the benefits. Just do what you know you can do!

This dovetails right into the **Power of Simple Daily Habits**. The quality of your health is a reflection of the little things you do consistently, whether they're good or bad. You can change the course of your health forever by simply adding a few simple, yet powerful daily habits. It doesn't take a huge shift. Making a small commitment can put the ball in motion.

I mean daily habits like 10 minutes of rebounding in the morning and 5 minutes of deep breathing before bed. Dry brushing before the shower, using almond milk instead of cow's milk, making soups a vital few times a week for dinner. Bringing lunch from home a few times a week.

Combining 80/20 with Simple Daily Habits is twice as powerful!

You've just given yourself a fresh start by doing the ARC, so by maintaining a vital few of its simple daily habits, you can make your new health a reality for the rest of your life, month upon month, and year upon year.

Of course, no one, not I or anyone else, can promise you perfect health for the rest of your life. But you can stack the deck in your favor with good nutrition and lifestyle choices. And you can improve the quality of your daily life by giving yourself the tools for the energy and vitality to enjoy it.

I fully understand and appreciate that part of the joy of life is food and drink, socializing, entertaining, celebrating, and trying new, exciting things. I indulge, just like everyone else! But by sticking with a few core, consistent actions and locking these in as daily habits, you will build a foundation that will amplify your Cleanse benefits tenfold.

FOUR CORE ACTIONS

If you do nothing else, take these Four Core Actions as you go forth from Day Zero. They are the epitome of putting in minimum effort to get the maximum benefit. Each action literally requires 0.4 percent of your time each week but will give you a whole new level of health without needing to make a *major* lifestyle change.

It's about keeping it honest, together, and applying the philosophy of simplicity and fun. That's what I'm about (and what life should be about).

Core Action #1: Daily Juice or Smoothie

Over the past week you've juiced and made smoothies and soups every day. By now, you're amazing at it, and have the process *down*. And that's one of the biggest gifts of the ARC! You've learned all the shortcuts, your taste preferences, and just how easy it is.

So keep it going. **Make an alkaline juice or smoothie every day.**

You don't need to make it fresh every day. You can stick with your routine of making twice the volume you need, and storing the second serving for next time. At this rate, you'll make juices or smoothies only three or four times a week max. You have 10,080 minutes in a week, so this is only 0.4 percent of your time. You can certainly manage that!

I strive for five to seven servings of fresh greens every day, a life-changing habit made easy with one daily juice or smoothie. You can get almost all of them into just that one drink! Juicing/making smoothies also gives you a chance to get in a wonderful variety of Triple A foods, including anti-inflammatory turmeric, ginger, garlic, and antioxidants like carrots, bell peppers, and beets.

Once you stick with it for a few more days, you will stick with it for life. Why? When you *don't* have your daily juice or smoothie, you'll really feel the difference!

Core Action #2: Proper Hydration

You've worked hard to get your hydration up to 100 ounces (or more) per day via herbal teas, turmeric teas, and filtered water. By now, it's already part of your routine. Keep it up! **Continue having three to four liters of water every day to stay super-hydrated.** This alone can be life- and health-changing for most people.

It takes about five minutes per day to physically drink that water, another 40 minutes per week, or another 0.4 percent of your time.

If you haven't already, you can upgrade from filtered water to alkaline water. You can make yourself dizzy researching all the options in faucet-attached alkaline filters, countertop pitchers, drops, etc. For now, getting a decent countertop pitcher is a good start.

Core Action #3: Daily Healthy Fats

It takes a little focus, and a small amount of effort, to get enough healthy fats each day. As a reminder, the amount to shoot for is three tablespoons of omega 3 and one tablespoon of coconut oil each day. You've been doing it. Just keep on doing it.

Please don't fear these fats! They will not make you gain weight. They will increase your metabolism and lower bad cholesterol, lube up your digestion, and improve brain and skin health. They give your body excellent fuel.

Stock up on healthy oils; look for ways to incorporate flax oil, coconut oil, nuts, and seeds into your meals every day; and keep taking the supplements. Another five-minute (or less) a day task, and another 0.4 percent of your week's time.

Core Action #4: Movement

I say "movement" vs. "exercise" because everyone has such personal preferences about fitness. Some might love it and exercise daily with a variety of sports and regimens. Others can't stand it, haven't had a regimen for years, if ever, and would rather poke out their eyes than hit the gym. I am not going to tell you the type of exercise you *have* to do, but I heartily recommend that you simply *move* every day.

Moving gets your heart rate going to make you aerobically strong. Exercise resistance strengthens bones, too. It uses your muscles, pumps your lymph and blood, revs your metabolism, and helps clear toxins. Just imagine metabolic waste products and toxins in a stagnant pool inside your body. All it takes to get them out is a nice walk, some time on the mini-tramp, a yoga class, a run, or a little circuit of push-ups and squats in your bedroom—*anything*.

It's imperative you do *something* every day, even if it's just for a minimum amount of eight minutes. It clears your mind and helps you sleep better, wake earlier, and feel more energized throughout the day. In effect, exercise gives you back time you would have spent tired or zoned out, so I don't calculate it as time spent since it actually adds hours to your week.

As with everything I coach, movement should be simple and fun. If it were painful and hard, you wouldn't do it! Keep your body flowing and your energy pumping. If you raise your heart rate a little, sweat a little, or use your muscles a little, you've won the day.

One Golden Rule for Day Zero

My one golden rule for Day Zero: Don't have a blowout celebration meal!

On Day Zero, you are facing a huge opportunity. It would be a massive shame to celebrate that opportunity by going out and having pizza, ice cream, beer, or all the things that have been "missing." Rewarding oneself with the things you know are harmful is a slippery slope on many levels. Emotionally, it's the opposite of practicing self-love. Neurologically, it activates the brain's pleasure/reward center with a damaging substance (*exactly* like drug abuse). Hormonally, it triggers a chemical cascade that will make it almost impossible for you to resist cravings for more junk food.

You don't need to totally restrict yourself on Day Zero. You just need to reward yourself with something wonderful, extravagant, *and* healthful. And it will be pretty easy to do. Having been through seven days of self-care and goodness, you'll feel *so* in tune with your body that you won't even crave those blowout foods and beverages anymore. The less sugar, wheat, processed foods, and meat you eat, the less you will want. The more good stuff you take in, the more you'll have a taste for it.

Another big benefit I've noticed is that the Cleanse week effectively toggles a mental switch. You learn that positive rewards come from positive actions. In the past, you may have had a habit of seeking positive rewards (feeling good, comfort) from negative actions (substance abuse, emotional eating, etc.). The Cleanse resets that impulse, and the last thing you need is to revert to the behavior that threw your body out of balance in the first place.

So what should you eat and drink this weekend? It will come as no surprise to you that I have a created a plan for that.

Day Zero

On Day Zero, it's all about easing yourself back into solid foods and "normal" eating while continuing with some Cleanse-brought changes. I strongly recommend keeping the habit of lemon water and one of the turmeric tea recipes going for life. You don't have to do it *every* day but try to have the lemon water as often as possible first thing and the turmeric every other day.

A "normal" breakfast is called for today. Chewing! Remember that? I have given you a few delicious, different options throughout the Cleanse, but I love to kick off Day Zero with the Super Nutrient Breakfast Bowl. It's warm, cooked, texture-rich, flavor-rich, and super alkaline. It's a great way to get at least one juice in on Day Zero, and if you're making one, you may as well make two servings so you can have a second one later in the day.

Definitely think ahead to snacks and prepare your old friend from prep week, Easy Bliss Balls (page 120), or this new recipe for Alkaline Superfood Balls. They are both great options because you can make the whole batch and store in the fridge until you're ready to eat. Or you can freeze them and let thaw for two hours before eating. Another snack option is my hummus recipe with vegetable sticks or gluten-free crackers.

Aside from that, feel free to have whatever else you would like to eat for lunch and dinner. Just have a side salad with each meal, and you're all set.

Day Zero Meal Plan

Upon rising: Lemon water, Turmeric and Ginger Refresher Tea
Prebreakfast: Triple A Juice (page 64)
Breakfast: Super-Nutrient Breakfast Bowl (page 118)
Lunch: Anything you like with a big side salad!
Midafternoon snack: Triple A Juice *or* Alkaline Superfood Balls *or* Alkaline Creamy Hummus and Vegetable Sticks
Dinner: Anything you like with a big side salad!

ALKALINE SUPERFOOD BALLS

Makes 5 servings (3 balls per serving)

Ingredients

½ cup almonds
⅓ cup pepitas (pumpkin seeds)
⅓ cup walnuts
¼ cup black sesame seeds

⅓ cup chia seeds
¼ cup almond butter
½ cup tahini
¼ cup coconut palm sugar

Instructions

Simply blend all the ingredients and roll into balls!

ALKALINE CREAMY HUMMUS AND VEGETABLE STICKS

Makes 4 servings

Ingredients

For the hummus

1 12-ounce can chickpeas
1 tablespoon tahini paste
1 garlic clove, finely chopped or crushed

Juice of ½ lemon
1 tablespoon olive oil
Salt and pepper to taste

Crudités

Sticks of celery, carrots, bell peppers, cucumbers (whatever your heart—and stomach—desires)

Instructions

Blend the hummus ingredients, place in bowl, and scoop with veggie sticks.

Day Zero, Again

Every day from now on is Day Zero. You aren't counting up and down, you are just alive, eating well, and enjoying life! The only things I want you to count from now on are glasses of water and your breaths while meditating. If the second day post-Cleanse for you is Sunday, you have all day long to enjoy how great you feel and to make some wonderful recipes . . .

Day Zero, Again, Meal Plan

Upon rising: Lemon water, Creamy Turmeric and Coconut Tea (page 159)

Breakfast: Alkaline Baked Bean Salsa Brekkie (that's Australian for "breakfast," mate)

Midmorning snack: Live Energized Green Juice (page 155)

Lunch: Anything you like with a big side salad!

Midafternoon snack: Live Energized Green Juice *or* Alkaline Superfood Balls *or* Alkaline Creamy Hummus and Vegetable Sticks

Dinner: Anything you like with a big side salad!

ALKALINE BAKED BEAN SALSA BREKKIE

Makes 2 servings

Ingredients

2 garlic cloves, finely chopped

6 cherry tomatoes, halved

1 12-ounce can haricot beans (or lentils, kidney beans, black beans, adzuki beans, all preferably organic)

4 scallions, roughly chopped

1 handful of basil

2 handfuls of spinach

Himalayan salt and black pepper, to taste

½ teaspoon coconut oil

1 avocado, halved

Juice from ½ lemon

Olive oil

Instructions

Boil ¼ cup water in a frying pan and "steam fry" the garlic for 1 minute. Throw in the cherry tomatoes, beans, and scallions and cook until everything softens.

Add the basil and spinach. Cook until wilted and season with Himalayan salt and black pepper. Stir in the coconut oil.

Serve the bean salsa with a halved avocado with lemon juice and olive oil drizzled all over.

THE ONLY RECIPE YOU'LL EVER NEED

Of course, I've given you several recipes throughout the Cleanse, and you can find hundreds of Triple A recipes on my website, including lots of extra "After the ARC" recipes for breakfast, lunch, dinner, juices, smoothies, soups, and snacks. But if you want to just wing it yourself, every recipe you make should be based on these two instructions:

1. Keep it simple.

2. Add more good stuff.

After the ARC, you'll be super-motivated to keep going, and it's important that you don't make things too complicated or perfect. You don't need to go from finishing the Cleanse to living a life of perfection.

Remember, perfection isn't the aim.

You *will* feel amazing, and this will be incredibly motivating to you to make smart, healthier decisions when you're at crossroads throughout the day. When your workmate brings through the cookie jar, you'll naturally feel more likely to say no. When you are out for dinner, instead of choosing the cheesy pasta dish, you'll be more likely to go for the grilled salmon with vegetables. When it comes to soda or water, you'll just feel more like choosing the water.

Your body will feel so good that you won't want to undo that feeling. You will start to think, *Well, I could have that cookie, but it's just not worth it.* These types of conflicts will be likely, but your decisions will become automatic. Eventually, the entire conversations will be subconscious.

However, there is no pressure. Let yourself relax, and for the first few weeks after the ARC, focus your energy on cooking simply (and therefore, making it more likely you'll make your own food, a huge positive for your health), and adding more good stuff. Outside of that, worry less about cutting stuff out, but rather keep on thinking about what you can add in. When you use this approach, you are letting your brain decide when you're ready to progress. You can stop thinking about it entirely!

My "Crowd Out the Bad" Method for Lifelong, Easy, Abundant Health

The more good stuff you add in, and the more alkaline, balanced, and healthy you get, the more alkaline, balanced, and healthy you *will* get. It's like how the "rich get richer." You can start as slowly as you like with this approach because the best part is, as you add good stuff, you *naturally* remove the bad stuff.

Both your conscious and subconscious minds will help you do this. This is the process that builds upon everything I've just discussed. It is the epitome of Pareto's Principle applied to your health alongside the power of habits. It's the training that all of my Alkaline Reset Cleanse clients go through in our After the Cleanse training, and the very first thing that all of my Alkaline Base Camp members go through too. You can start as slowly as you like with this approach because the best part is, as you add good stuff, you *naturally* remove the bad stuff.

Both your conscious and subconscious minds will help you do this.

Consciously, you will feel better. You'll think, *I like this! I'm going to do what I know will continue this good feeling.* You will *want* to make the right choice. After a few days, weeks, or months, you will find yourself *wanting* to say no to certain foods or drinks because you will feel so great, you won't want to change that. You'll get more picky with your treats and save your blowouts for social events that matter rather than a casual random dessert or bottle of wine.

Subconsciously, your below-the-surface mind will have been very busy learning new things. It's a fast learner and will work out that the longer you live energized, the better you will feel and the sharper you will be. Your brain will put two and two together and notice that action equals positive response in your body. Your subconscious will *want* you to keep doing what supports its functioning. It will send the message to your conscious mind, "More healthy fats! More plant proteins! More hydration!" And you will find yourself reaching for the coconut oil and water pitcher. Your brain will become your "healthy filter." You'll stop noticing temptations or being drawn toward them.

Have you ever been in a good healthy place in your mind where when you are at the grocery store, as you head down the freezer aisle, you are so focused on getting to the healthy section that you don't even see the ice cream? That was your brain filtering *for* you.

Let your subconscious drive the bus, with your conscious mind pointing out roadside attractions. When you make healthier choices on autopilot, you don't need willpower and won't experience anxiety and stress. You will gradually become more alkaline, healthy, and energized while going about your business. My clients and I go really deep on this in the program, and because I want you to really understand and get the most out of this, I have included some of our deep-dive training in the Resources so you can make sure you get the benefit from this powerful approach.

I believe that what you bring into your life and your body determines whether you'll be happy and successful. If you want joy and vitality, bring in people and foods that are going to support you in that goal. The more good stuff you bring into your body, the more likely you will be successful in your relationships and career. It all starts with you and how you treat yourself. As you connect these dots—good food → better health → more vitality → clearer mind → less stress → happier relationships → better ideas → the energy to achieve goals—you will understand how fundamental this is for overall success and happiness.

You and your body are a team, so work together for your greater good. Balance is the key and the only way to feel as good as you can.

This is how to live, for life.

This is the way you want to feel forever.

You will never want to lose this feeling—and you never have to.

Live energized, now and forever.

RESOURCES

Alkaline-Forming Foods	
Vegetables	
Asparagus	Garlic
Basil	Green Beans
Beetroot	Kale
Broad Beans	Kelp
Broccoli	Lettuce
Brussels sprouts	Onion
Cabbage	Parsley
Carrot	Peas
Cauliflower	Pepper/Capsicum
Celery	Pumpkin
Chard	Radish
Chili peppers	Runner Beans
Chinese cabbage/Wombok	Snowpeas
Chives	Spinach
Collards	String Beans
Coriander/Cilantro	Sweet Potato
Cucumber	Wakame
Dandelion	Watercress
Eggplant/Aubergine	Zucchini/Courgette
Endive	

Fruit	
Avocado	Lemon
Coconut	Lime
Grapefruit	Tomato

* Lower sugar berries are the best of the rest, including strawberries, blueberries, and raspberries.

Nuts and Seeds	
Almonds	Hazelnuts
Cashews	Macadamia nuts
Chia Seeds	Pumpkin seeds
Coconut	Sesame seeds
Flax Seeds	Sunflower seeds

Sprouts	
Alfalfa sprouts	Fenugreek sprouts
Amaranth sprouts	Soy sprouts
Barley grass	Wheatgrass
Broccoli sprouts	* Any other sprout

Breads	
Gluten/yeast-free breads and wraps	Sprouted wraps
Sprouted bread	

Grains, Beans, and Pulses	
Amaranth	Navy beans
Brown rice	Pinto beans
Buckwheat	Quinoa
Lentils	Red beans
Lima Beans	Soy beans
Millet	White beans
Mung beans	

Oils	
Avocado oil	MCT oils
Coconut oil	Olive oil
Flax oil	Pumpkin seed oil

Spices	
Cardamom	Ginger
Cinnamon	Turmeric
Cloves	
Other	
Alkaline water	Oily, wild-caught fish (in moderation)
Herbal teas	

Acid-Forming Foods

Meat	
Bacon	Pork
Beef	Rabbit
Corned Beef	Turkey
Lamb	Veal
Organ Meats	Venison
Seafood	
Clams	Oysters
Lobster	Prawns
Other crustaceans	
Fruits (should be kept to 1-2 servings per day)	
Apple	Orange
Apricot	Peach
Berries	Pear
Cantaloupe	Pineapple
Cranberries	Plum
Dried fruit	Raspberries
Grapes	Strawberries
Mango	Tropical fruits
Melon	

Dairy	
Cheese	Milk
Eggs	Sour Cream
Ice Cream	
Drinks	
Alcohol	Diet drinks
Black tea	Energy drinks
Carbonated water	Flavored water
Cocoa	Fruit juice
Coffee	Green tea
Colas	Sports drinks
Dairy milk	Tap water
Decaffeinated drinks	
Sweeteners and Sugars	
Agave syrup	Date syrup
Any refined sugar	Fructose
Artificial sweeteners	High fructose corn syrup
Carob	Honey
Coconut syrup	Maple syrup
Corn syrup	Molasses
Fats and Oils	
Any cooked oil (except coconut)	Safflower
Canola	Solid oils (margarine)
Other Omega–6-rich vegetable oils	Sunflower
Partially or fully hydrogenated oils	
Condiments	
Ketchup	Store-bought sauces
Mayonnaise	Tabasco
Pickles	Vinegar
Soy Sauce	

Other	
Gluten (wheat, spelt, rye, and barley)	Natural and Artificial Colors
Monosodium glutamate	Natural and Artificial Flavors
Mushrooms	Vinegars

For the full Acid/Alkaline Food Chart go to Your ARC Resources at www.rossbridgeford.com/arc.

SHOPPING LISTS

Shopping List for Days One, Two, and Three

Greens, Herbs, and Other Veggies

Arugula	1 bag or 2 bunches
Avocado	5
Beet	2
Broccoli	1 large head
Cabbage, Chinese	1 head
Carrot	7
Celery	10 stalks
Chard	1 bunch
Cilantro	1 bunch
Cucumber	7
Dill	1 bunch
Garlic	1 bulb
Kale	2 big bunches
Leek	1
Lettuce	1 head
Onion, yellow	2
Pepper, green	1
Pepper, red	3
Squash, butternut	1
Spinach	5 bags or 10 bunches
Sweet potato	1
Tomato	3

Roots

Galangal	2-inch root
Ginger	1 large root
Turmeric	2 large roots (or 5 small)

Citrus

Lemon	3
Lime	1

Seasonings

Cayenne	1 jar
Black pepper	1 jar/grinder
Nutmeg	1 small jar
Himalayan salt	1 jar/grinder
Sea salt	1 jar/grinder
Vanilla pod (optional)	1

Oils

Coconut oil	1 jar
Olive oil	1 small bottle

Legumes

Lentils, dry	2 cups

Nuts and Seeds

Almonds (raw, unsalted)	4 ounces
Cashews (raw, unsalted)	6 ounces
Chia seeds	3 ounces
Sunflower seeds	6 ounces

Liquids

Almond milk	2 quarts
Coconut milk	2 16-ounce cans
Coconut water	1 quart
Vegetable stock	3.5 quarts

Shopping List for Days Four through Seven

Greens, Herbs, and Other Veggies

Avocado	4
Beet	1
Broccoli	8 heads
Cabbage, white	1 head
Carrots	7
Celery	8 stalks
Cilantro	1 large bunch
Cucumber	10
Garlic	1 bulb
Kale	2 bunches
Kale, Tuscan	1 bunch
Lettuce	1 head
Mint	1 bunch
Onion, red	2
Onion, yellow	1
Parsley, flat-leaf	1 bunch
Pepper, red	3
Potato, red bliss	1
Pumpkin	2 12-ounce cans (or 1 small)
Squash, butternut	1
Scallion	2 bunches
Spinach	5 bags or 10 bunches
Tomato	10
Watercress	3 bunches

Roots

Ginger	1 large root
Turmeric	3 large roots (or 7 small)

Citrus

Lemon	4
Lime	1

Seasonings

Cumin	1 jar
Mustard seeds	1 jar

Legumes

Cannellini beans (canned)	4 cups
Lentils, dry	1 cup

Liquids

Coconut cream	1 12-ounce can
Coconut milk	2 12-ounce cans
Coconut water	2 liters
Vegetable stock	3 liters

RECIPE LIST

TEAS AND TONICS

Creamy Turmeric and Coconut Tea (p. 159)
Digestive Tea (p. 122)
Turmeric and Coconut Tea (p. 118)
Turmeric and Ginger Refresher Tea (p. 155)

JUICES

Alkaline High-Energy Juice (p. 159)
Alkaline Immune-Boosting Juice (p. 136)
Anti-Inflammation Juice (p. 162)
Blood-Builder Juice (p. 168)
Digestion Juice (p. 169)
Live Energized Green Juice (p. 155)
Triple A Juice (p. 64)

SMOOTHIES

Alkaline Avocado Power Smoothie (p. 160)
All-Day Energy Smoothie (p. 162)
Anti-Inflammatory Smoothie (p. 170)
Antioxidant Green Smoothie (p. 119)
Core Green Alkaline Smoothie (p. 156)

Soups

Meals

Snacks

CONVERSION CHART

Standard Cup	Fine Powder (e.g., flour)	Grain (e.g., rice)	Granular (e.g., sugar)	Liquid Solids (e.g., butter)	Liquid (e.g., milk)
1	140 g	150 g	190 g	200 g	240 ml
¾	105 g	113 g	143 g	150 g	180 ml
⅔	93 g	100 g	125 g	133 g	160 ml
1/2	70 g	75 g	95 g	100 g	120 ml
⅓	47 g	50 g	63 g	67 g	80 ml
¼	35 g	38 g	48 g	50 g	60 ml
⅛	18 g	19 g	24 g	25 g	30 ml

Useful Equivalents for Liquid Ingredients by Volume				
¼ tsp				1 ml
½ tsp				2 ml
1 tsp				5 ml
3 tsp	1 tbsp		½ fl oz	15 ml
	2 tbsp	⅛ cup	1 fl oz	30 ml
	4 tbsp	¼ cup	2 fl oz	60 ml
	5⅓ tbsp	⅓ cup	3 fl oz	80 ml
	8 tbsp	½ cup	4 fl oz	120 ml
	10⅔ tbsp	⅔ cup	5 fl oz	160 ml
	12 tbsp	¾ cup	6 fl oz	180 ml
	16 tbsp	1 cup	8 fl oz	240 ml
	1 pt	2 cups	16 fl oz	480 ml
	1 qt	4 cups	32 fl oz	960 ml
			33 fl oz	1000 ml 1 L

Useful Equivalents for Dry Ingredients by Weight		
(To convert ounces to grams, multiply the number of ounces by 30.)		
1 oz	1/16 lb	30 g
4 oz	¼ lb	120 g
8 oz	½ lb	240 g
12 oz	¾ lb	360 g
16 oz	1 lb	480 g

Useful Equivalents for Cooking/Oven Temperatures			
Process	Fahrenheit	Celsius	Gas Mark
Freeze Water	32° F	0° C	
Room Temperature	68° F	20° C	
Boil Water	212° F	100° C	
Bake	325° F	160° C	3
	350° F	180° C	4
	375° F	190° C	5
	400° F	200° C	6
	425° F	220° C	7
	450° F	230° C	8
Broil			Grill

Useful Equivalents for Length				
(To convert inches to centimeters, multiply the number of inches by 2.5.)				
1 in			2.5 cm	
6 in	½ ft		15 cm	
12 in	1 ft		30 cm	
36 in	3 ft	1 yd	90 cm	
40 in			100 cm	1 m

ENDNOTES

Chapter 1: How Did We Get Here?

1. Chatterjee et al., "Chronic Disease and Wellness in America: Measuring the Economic Burden of a Changing Nation," Milken Institute (January 2014).

2. "Obesity Update," Organisation for Economic Co-Operation and Development (OECD) (2014).

3. "National Diabetes Statistics Report, 2017: Estimates of Diabetes and Its Burden in the United States," Centers for Disease Control and Prevention (July 2017).

4. Lenoir et al., "Intense Sweetness Surpasses Cocaine Reward," *PLOS One* (August 2007).

5. Chowdhury et al., "Association of dietary, circulating, and supplement fatty acids with coronary risk: a systematic review and meta-analysis," *Annals of Internal Medicine* (March 2014).

6. Mak Daulatzai, "Non-celia gluten sensitivity triggers gut dysbiosis, neuroinflammation, gut-brain axis dysfunction, and vulnerability for dementia," *CNS & Neurological Disorders - Drug Targets* (2015).

7. Soares et al., "Gluten-free diet reduces adiposity, inflammation, and insulin resistance associated with the induction of PPAR-alpha and PPAR-gamma expression," *Journal of Nutritional Biochemistry* (June 2013).

8. Karin de Punder and Leo Pruimboom, "The Dietary Intake of Wheat and other Cereal Grains and Their Role in Inflammation," *Nutrients* (March 2013).

9. Lammers et al., "Gliadin induces an increase in intestinal permeability and zonulin release by binding to the chemokine receptor CXCR3," *Gastroenterology* (July 2008).

10. Richard C. Shelton and Andrew H. Miller, "Eating ourselves to death (and despair): The contribution of adiposity and inflammation to depression," *Progress in Neurobiology* (August 2010).

11. Preetha Anaud, "Cancer is a preventable disease that requires major lifestyle changes," *Pharmaceutical Research* (September 2008).

12. "Simple Steps to Preventing Diabetes," Harvard T.H. Chan School of Public Health's The Nutrition Source.

13. Howard LeWine, M.D., "200,000 Heart Disease, Stroke Deaths a Year Are Preventable," Harvard Health Publishing (September 2013).

14. "Preventing Stroke: Healthy Living," Centers for Disease Control and Prevention and Health Promotion (January 2017).

15. "Prevention and Risk of Alzheimer's and Dementia," Alzheimer's Association Research Center (2018).

Chapter 2: The Five Master Systems

1. Foster-Powell et al., "International table of glycemic index and glycemic load values," *American Journal of Clinical Nutrition* (July 2002).

2. Maurer et al., "Neutralization of Western diet inhibits bone resorption independently of K intake and reduces cortisol secretion in humans," *American Journal of Physiology-Renal Physiology* (September 2002).

3. Gaggl et al., "Effect of oral alkali supplementation on progression of chronic kidney disease," *Current Hypertension Reviews* (2014).

4. de Brito-Ashurst et al., "Bicarbonate supplementation slows progression of CKD and improves nutritional status," *Journal of the American Society of Nephrology* (September 2009).

Chapter 3: Your Body's Number-One Goal

1. Williams et al., "The role of dietary acid load and mild metabolic acidosis in insulin resistance in humans," *Biochimie* (May 2016).

2. Fagherazzi et al., "Dietary acid load and risk of type 2 diabetes: the E3N-EPIC cohort study," *Diabetologia* (February 2014).

3. Carnauba et al., "Diet-Induced Low-Grade Metabolic Acidosis and Clinical Outcomes: A Review," *Nutrients* (May 2017).

4. Julia Scialla, "The balance of the evidence on acid-base homeostasis and progression of chronic kidney disease," *Kidney International* (May 2015).

5. Dawson-Hughes et al., "Alkaline diets favor lean tissue mass in older adults," *American Journal of Clinical Nutrition* (March 2008).

6. Ian Forrest Robey, "Examining the relationship between diet-induced acidosis and cancer," *Nutrition & Metabolism* (August 2012).

7. Jehle et al., "Partial neutralization of the acidogenic Western diet with potassium citrate increases bone mass in postmenopausal women with osteopenia," *Journal of the American Society of Nephrology: JASN* (November 2006).

8. Ian Forrest Robey, "Examining the relationship between diet-induced acidosis and cancer," *Nutrition & Metabolism* (August 2012).

9. Whitworth et al., "Cardiovascular consequences of cortisol excess," *Vascular Health and Risk Management* (December 2005).

10. David Allen Bushinsky, M.D., "Acid-base imbalance and the skeleton," *European Journal of Nutrition* (October 2001).

11. Caroline Passey, "Reducing the Dietary Acid Load: How a More Alkaline Diet Benefits Patients with Chronic Kidney Disease," *Journal of Renal Nutrition* (May 2017).

Chapter 4: The Top Three Imbalancers

1. Yong-Moon Park et al., "High dietary acid load is associated with risk of breast cancer: findings from the Sister Study," *The FASEB Journal* (April 2017).

2. Park et al., "Association between the markers of metabolic acid load and higher all-cause and cardiovascular mortality in a general population with preserved renal function," *Journal of Hypertension Research* (March 2015).

3. Zhang et al., "Consumption of fruits and vegetables and risk of renal cell carcinoma: a meta-analysis of observational studies," *Oncotarget* (April 2017).

4. Ribeiro et al., "Buffer therapy for cancer," *Journal of Nutrition & Food Sciences* (April 2012).

5. Park et al., "Association between the markers of metabolic acid load and higher all-cause and cardiovascular mortality in a general population with preserved renal function," *Journal of Hypertension Research* (March 2015).

6. Teta et al., "Acidosis downregulates leptin production from cultured adipocytes through a glucose transport-dependent post-transcriptional mechanism," *Journal of the American Society of Nephrology* (June 2003).

7. Disthabanchong et al., "Metabolic acidosis lowers circulating adiponectin through inhibition of adiponectin gene transcription," *Nephrology Dialysis Transplantation* (July 2010).

8. Robert C. Andrews and Brian R. Walker, "Glucocorticoids and insulin resistance: old hormones, new targets," *Clinical Science* (May 1999).

9. Brüngger et al., "Effect of chronic metabolic acidosis on thyroid hormone homeostasis in humans," *American Journal of Physiology* (May 1997).

10. Bahrami et al., "Inflammatory Markers Associated with Subclinical Coronary Artery Disease: The Multicenter AIDS Cohort Study," *Journal of the American Heart Association* (June 2016).

11. Maximilian Zeyda and Thomas M. Stulnig, "Obesity, inflammation, and insulin resistance—a mini-review," *Gerontology* (April 2009).

12. Lim et al., "Peripheral inflammation and cognitive aging," *Modern Trends in Pharmacopsychiatry* (February 2013).

13. Karim et al., "Renal handling of NH4+ in relation to the control of acid-base balance by the kidney," *Journal of Nephrology* (March 2002).

14. Guyre et al., "Glucocorticoid effects on the production and actions of immune cytokines," *Journal of Steroid Biochemistry* (1988).

15. Keith N. Frayn, "Adipose tissue and the insulin resistance syndrome," *Proceedings of the Nutrition Society* (August 2001).

Chapter 5: Back in Balance with the Triple A Method

1. Pizzorno et al., "Diet-induced acidosis: is it real and clinically relevant?" *British Journal of Nutrition* (December 2009).

2. Sebastian et al., "Estimation of the net acid load of the diet of ancestral preagricultural Homo sapiens and their hominid ancestors," *American Journal of Clinical Nutrition* (December 2002).

3. Jennifer Di Noia, Ph.D., "Defining Powerhouse Fruits and Vegetables: A Nutrient Density Approach," *Preventing Chronic Disease* (2014).

4. Gerry K. Schwalfenberg, "The Alkaline Diet: Is There Evidence That an Alkaline pH Diet Benefits Health?" *Journal of Environmental and Public Health* (2012).

5. Belcaro et al., "Product-evaluation registry of Meriva®, a curcumin-phosphatidylcholine complex, for the complementary management of osteoarthritis," *Panminerva Medica* (June 2010).

6. Kailash Srivastava and Thikra Mustafa, "Ginger (Zingiber officinale) in rheumatism and musculoskeletal disorders," *Medical Hypotheses* (December 1992).

7. Zakaria et al., "In vivo Antinociceptive and Anti-inflammatory Activities of Dried and Fermented Processed Virgin Coconut Oil," *Medical Principles and Practice* (March 2011).

8. Ogbolu et al., "In vitro antimicrobial properties of coconut oil on Candida species in Ibadan, Nigeria," *Journal of Medicinal Food* (June 2007).

9. Vysakh et al., "Polyphenolics isolated from virgin coconut oil inhibits adjuvant induced arthritis in rats through antioxidant and anti-inflammatory action," *International Immunopharmacology* (May 2014).

10. Coleman et al., "Glaucoma risk and the consumption of fruits and vegetables among older women in the study of osteoporotic fractures," *American Journal of Ophthalmology* (June 2008).

11. Allen Y. Chen and Yi Charlie Chen, "A review of the dietary flavonoid, kaempferol on human health and cancer chemoprevention," *Food Chemistry* (June 2014).

12. Verhagen et al., "Reduction of oxidative DNA-damage in humans by brussels sprouts," *Carcinogenesis* (April 1995).

13. Geng et al., "Allyl isothiocyanate arrests cancer cells in mitosis, and mitotic arrest in turn leads to apoptosis via Bcl-2 protein phosphorylation," *Journal of Biological Chemistry* (September 2011).

Chapter 6: The Five Pillars of the ARC

1. National Research Council. "Fluoride in Drinking Water: A Scientific Review of EPA's Standards" (2006).

2. Choi et al., "Developmental Fluoride Neurotoxicity: A Systematic Review and Meta-Analysis," *Environmental Health Perspectives* (October 2012).

3. "Take Back the Tap: The Big Business Hustle of Bottled Water," Food & Water Watch (February 2018).

4. "State of American Drinking Water," Environmental Working Group (2018).

Chapter 8: Everything You'll Be Eating

1. Jennifer Di Noia, Ph.D., "Defining Powerhouse Fruits and Vegetables: A Nutrient Density Approach," *Preventing Chronic Disease* (2014).

2. Stanhope et al., "Consuming fructose-sweetened, not glucose-sweetened, beverages increases visceral adiposity and lipids and decreases insulin sensitivity in overweight/obese humans," *Journal of Clinical Investigation* (May 2009).

3. Bernadine Ruiza G. Ang and Gracia Fe Yu, "The Role of Fructose in Type 2 Diabetes and Other Metabolic Diseases," *Journal of Nutrition & Food Sciences* (January 2018).

4. DiNicolantonio et al., "Added Fructose," *Mayo Clinic Proceedings* (March 2015).

5. Robert P. Heaney and Connie M. Weaver, "Calcium absorption from kale," *American Journal of Clinical Nutrition* (January 1990).

6. Feskanich et al., "Milk, dietary calcium, and bone fractures in women: a 12-year prospective study," *American Journal of Public Health* (June 1997).

7. Sonneville et al., "Vitamin D, calcium, and dairy intakes and stress fractures among female adolescents," *Archives of Pediatrics & Adolescent Medicine* (July 2012).

Chapter 11: The Seven Days Before

1. Hall et al., "Sleep as a Mediator of the Stress-Immune Relationship," *Psychosomatic Medicine* (January 1998).

2. Ananthakrishnan et al., "Sleep disturbance and the risk of active disease in patients with Crohn's disease and ulcerative colitis," *Clinical Gastroenterology and Hepatology* (August 2013).

3. Xie et al., "Sleep drives metabolite clearance from the adult brain," *Science* (October 2013).

INDEX

ACKNOWLEDGMENTS

I first want to thank the love of my life and light of my life, Tania. Your ability to give me the truth when it's needed and unconditional love has made me a better man and father. You made this book possible. In fact, there would never have been a book without you.

To the amazing Valerie Frankel who is perhaps the best health editor in the World. I am still so honored at how much love, attention, and devotion you put into this project (you did the cleanse!). You took this to a whole other level with your skill, creativity, and ability to see all of my work and distill it to bring the most important messages to life. I am so thankful for you!

To the entire Hay House team, starting with Reid Tracy—you helped me believe in myself and gave me the guidance that only decades at the forefront of your field could bring. You have been incredibly generous. Patty Gift, you believed in me and gave me so much confidence in myself and this book.

To my Hay House editor Lisa Cheng, you have been so positive, supportive, and nurturing, and you somehow painlessly coerced me through my first external deadlines in 15 years with unbelievable ease and grace. Your ability as an editor is incredible, yet the level of understanding and support you gave was unexpected and hugely appreciated. There is always a smile on my face when we talk.

And to the amazing Hay House marketing and publicity team, in particular Lindsay McGinty, you have been a constant support and source of inspiration and ideas.

To Hay House Australia and Hay House UK, you have been so amazing along the way too. Special thanks to Leon Nacson and his beautiful team (and family) in Australia. You guys rock.

Thanks to Jeff Walker. You literally changed the course of my business and my life back in 2010 and I am so thankful to call you a friend eight years on. And, of course, to our whole Mastermind group who feels like my second family.

Huge gratitude to Ocean Robbins. You are always an inspiration, a wonderful support. Thank you, of course, for such a beautiful foreword to this book. And John Gallagher, you helped guide me through this process with calm and ease over multiple calls. And everyone else in Plat—all of you have helped me enormously in so many ways.

To my parents, Roger and Annette Bridgeford. Thank you for raising me in a supportive, loving environment, always encouraging me and believing in me and teaching me the importance of believing in myself. Dad, you have always shown me how important it is to be strong of mind and to take pride in what I do, and your humility and quiet strength have shaped who I am as a man. Mum, you have always led me to believe that I can only ever succeed, no matter the situation. Your love and support have helped me through so much. You both taught me how to think differently, and how to seek answers and ask questions. The love I have for you guys is infinite.

To my in-laws, Royston and Judy James. Thank you for everything you do to make me feel so loved here in Australia and for supporting all of us—myself, Tania, Leo, and Joe. We just love being around you both.

To my boys, Leo and Joe—you boys teach me something new about the world and about myself every day. You've also taught me that a whole new level of love exists.

And finally to my dog, Millie. When everything gets a bit too much, you just let me be me and remind me how simple it can be to be happy.

ABOUT THE AUTHOR

Ross Bridgeford is the creator of the Alkaline Reset Cleanse, Anti-Inflammation Breakthrough, and Alkaline Anti-Cancer Solution, as well as the Alkaline Diet Recipe Book series.

He has been teaching and coaching people to their biggest health, energy, and body goals for over 15 years, and he knows how to keep it simple and make it easy, effortless, and delicious.

Through rossbridgeford.com, he has reached over two million people a year, and through his programs, books, and courses, Ross has directly impacted the lives of over 10,000 clients from 64 different countries.

He lives in Brisbane, Australia, with his partner, Tania, and their two children.

Hay House Titles of Related Interest

YOU CAN HEAL YOUR LIFE, the movie, starring Louise Hay & Friends
(available as a 1-DVD program, an expanded 2-DVD set,
and an online streaming video)
Learn more at www.hayhouse.com/louise-movie

THE SHIFT, the movie, starring Dr. Wayne W. Dyer
(available as a 1-DVD program, an expanded 2-DVD set,
and an online streaming video)
Learn more at www.hayhouse.com/the-shift-movie

CULTURED FOOD IN A JAR: 100+ Probiotic Recipes to Inspire and Change Your Life,
by Donna Schwenk

*THE DENTAL DIET: The Surprising Link between Your Teeth, Real Food,
and Life-Changing Natural Health,* by Dr. Steven Lin

*FAT FOR FUEL: A Revolutionary Diet to Combat Cancer, Boost Brain Power,
and Increase Your Energy,* by Dr. Joseph Mercola

*FAT FOR FUEL KETOGENIC COOKBOOK: Recipes and Ketogenic Keys to Health
from a World-Class Doctor and an Internationally Renowned Chef,*
by Dr. Joseph Mercola and Pete Evans

All of the above are available at your local bookstore,
or may be ordered by contacting Hay House (see next page).

Free e-newsletters from Hay House, the Ultimate Resource for Inspiration

Be the first to know about Hay House's free downloads, special offers, giveaways, contests, and more!

 Get exclusive excerpts from our latest releases and videos from *Hay House Present Moments*.

 Our *Digital Products Newsletter* is the perfect way to stay up-to-date on our latest discounted eBooks, featured mobile apps, and Live Online and On Demand events.

 Learn with real benefits! *HayHouseU.com* is your source for the most innovative online courses from the world's leading personal growth experts. Be the first to know about new online courses and to receive exclusive discounts.

 Enjoy uplifting personal stories, how-to articles, and healing advice, along with videos and empowering quotes, within *Heal Your Life*.

 Have an inspirational story to tell and a passion for writing? Sharpen your writing skills with insider tips from *Your Writing Life*.

Sign Up Now!

Get inspired, educate yourself, get a complimentary gift, and share the wisdom!

Visit www.hayhouse.com/newsletters to sign up today!

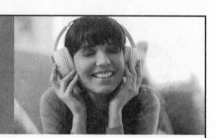